Medical Technology

Medical Technology
A nursing perspective

D.W. Hill

Regional Scientific Officer, North East Thames Regional Health Authority, UK
Visiting Professor in Biomedical Measurement, City University, London, UK

and

R. Summers

Lecturer in Systems Science, City University, London, UK

CHAPMAN & HALL
London · Glasgow · New York · Tokyo · Melbourne · Madras

**Published by Chapman & Hall, 2–6 Boundary Row,
London SE1 8HN, UK**

Chapman & Hall, 2–6 Boundary Row, London SE1 8HN, UK

Blackie Academic & Professional, Wester Cleddens Road,
Bishopbriggs, Glasgow G64 2NZ, UK

Chapman & Hall Inc., One Penn Plaza, 41st Floor,
New York NY10119, USA

Chapman & Hall Japan, Thomson Publishing Japan, Hirakawacho
Nemoto Building, 6F, 1-7-11 Hirakawa-cho, Chiyoda-ku, Tokyo 102,
Japan

Chapman & Hall Australia, Thomas Nelson Australia, 102 Dodds Street,
South Melbourne, Victoria 3205, Australia

Chapman & Hall India, R. Seshadri, 32 Second Main Road, CIT East,
Madras 600 035, India

Distributed in the USA and Canada by Singular Publishing Group Inc.
4284 41st Street, San Diego, California 92105

First edition 1994

© 1994 D. W. Hill and R. Summers

Typeset in Palatino 10½/12pt by Icon Graphic Services Ltd

Printed in Great Britain at The Alden Press, Oxford

ISBN 0 412 47090 X 1–56593–229–3 (USA)

A catalogue record for this book is available from the British Library

Library of Congress Catalog Card Number available

♾ Printed on permanent acid-free text paper, manufactured in accordance with ANSI/NISO Z39.48-1992 and ANSI/NISO Z39.48-1984
(Permanence of Paper).

Contents

Preface

High dependency environments in hospitals include intensive care units, special care baby units, operating and recovery rooms, coronary care units and burns units. The patients are in such a condition that they require a distinctly more intensive level of medical and nursing care than would be available in an ordinary ward. This level of care requires specially trained and experienced staff. It is likely that these will be available to a lesser degree than would be desired and thus it is important that reliable equipment is available to support them. While there is no substitute for devoted care by staff for patients, monitoring equipment can provide reliable visual, and often hard copy, recording of trends over extended periods without fatiguing staff and can accurately control infusions and ventilation.

The general availability of on-board computing power from a microcomputer is making medical instrumentation systems increasingly 'intelligent' and is leading to the application of knowledge-based systems for decision support in high dependency areas. There is a general desire by those charged with making patient-management decisions to have more robust data available and the collection of this and its reduction to sensible proportions is progressing steadily because of advances in technology.

Nurses in intensive care situations find themselves working with a wide range of technologies and, out of normal working hours, they may find themselves very much on their own. The purpose of this book is to introduce them to the basic principles involved and to illustrate typical applications. It is written firmly with the requirements of the user in mind and it is always pointed out that assistance should be sought where necessary from clinical engineers, applications specialists and service engineers.

Quite apart from a close involvement with life-support and patient-monitoring equipment, nurses may also find themselves assisting with the use and disinfection of sophisticated devices such as electronic endoscopy systems where mishandling can prove to be expensive in terms of repair or replacement.

There is a danger in writing a book on such a wide-ranging topic as 'Medical Technology', of being caught in the trap of endeavouring to include virtually every aspect of technology employed in high dependency situations. The authors have deliberately limited the scope of this book to subjects encompassed within their experience and where nurses are likely to be significantly involved, rather than those in which they are observers of the technology although providing nursing care for the patients concerned.

It is a pleasure to acknowledge the invaluable advice and assistance offered by staff, postgraduate students and members of courses for biomedical engineers and intensive care nurses at the City University and colleagues at the North East Thames Regional Health Authority and numerous hospitals, together with technical information and details of clinical applications from a number of major manufacturers and their sales staff and service engineers.

Glossary of Terms

ACCELERATION   Time rate of change of velocity e.g. metres per second per second

ACID   A substance which can donate hydrogen ions

ADC   Analogue-to-digital converter. A device which converts analogue data to digital form

ADDRESS   The identification of a specific location in a source of data or a computer's memory

ALGORITHM   An unambiguous series of steps leading to the solution of a problem

ANALOGUE   A signal or data which varies in a continuous fashion

ARTIFACT   A feature not naturally present, introduced during collection or processing

ASCII   American national standard code for information exchange. The standard code used to represent control characters, letters, numbers and graphics in data-processing systems

BANDWIDTH   The range of frequencies with defined upper and lower limits between which a system operates

BASE   A substance which can accept hydrogen ions. All soluble bases are alkaline substances

BIT   Contraction of 'binary digit', the smallest unit of data held in a computer (usually 0 or 1)

BUFFER   An area of storage which is reserved for use in performing an input/output operation into which data are written or from which data are read

BUFFER SOLUTION   A substance which minimizes any change in pH when either acid or base is added to a solution containing the buffer

BUS   Contraction of 'busbar'. One or more conductors used for transmitting signals or power

BYTE   A group of binary characters operated upon as a unit and usually shorter than a computer word, e.g. an 8-bit byte

cc   cubic centimetres, a measure of volume. (Not an SI unit of measurement. This has been replaced by the SI unit, cm^3.)

CCD   Charge coupled device. An imaging chip whose development has been important in the development of fibre optic endoscopes

CCU   Coronary care unit

CLOSED LOOP CONTROL   A control system in which decisions on actions are taken automatically on the basis of data collected from the patient

COMMUNICATIONS PORT   The provision in a computer to accommodate a data-communication device

COMPATIBILITY   The basic ability of different items of equipment to work together, taking into account the subtleties of their interaction

CPU   Central processing unit. The part of a computer which controls the interpretation and execution of instructions

CRT   Cathode ray tube e.g. a television picture tube used to display images or alphanumerical data

DATA COMPRESSION   A technique for reducing the required data-storage capacity by storing data in encoded form to eliminate gaps, empty fields and redundancies

DIGITAL   The representation of data or physical variables in the form of discrete numerical values

DAC   Digital-to-analogue converter. A device which converts digital data to analogue form

DECIBEL (dB)   A logarithmic unit to express current, power or voltage ratios measured across a specified resistance or impedance

DIGITIZE   To transcribe an analogue signal into digital form, usually for subsequent use by computer-processing methods. For example, an analogue time signal (hands on a clock face) must be converted to a digital time signal before it can be stored in computer memory

DIN   German standards body responsible for the specification of a popular range of plugs and sockets

DISK   A flat circular plate having a special surface to store data in digital form, e.g. floppy disk, hard disk, optical disk

DISTORTION   Any unwanted deviation from the original signal

DOPPLER SHIFT   Shift in frequency of a beam of sound or ultrasound on striking a moving reflector

DUPLEX   In data communications a full duplex arrangement allows one way at a time independent transmission

DYNAMIC RANGE   The ratio in decibels between the greatest and the smallest amplitudes of signal which a particular system or component can handle within quoted limits of linearity

ECG   Electrocardiogram. Electrical signal generated by the beating heart and normally initiated by the spontaneous activity of the natural cardiac pacemaker

EEG   Electroencephalogram. Signal generated by the electrical activity of the brain

EMF   The open-circuit (no-load) voltage produced by an electrochemical cell or battery. Its value depends on the nature of the chemicals employed

EMF   Electromotive force. Voltage supplied by a signal source or power supply under no-load (open-circuit) conditions

EMG   Electromyogram. Signal generated by the electrical activity of muscle

EHT   Extra high tension: the high voltage applied to cathode ray tubes or the capacitor of a defibrillator

FAULT TOLERANT   A system in which the failure of components does not cause the system to fail. Back-up components are available for automatic activation if the primary component fails

FIBRE OPTIC   A two-component flexible glass fibre made from an inner core of glass having a higher refractive index than the outer cladding. Light is transmitted efficiently down the core via a series of total internal reflections

FILTER   An electrical circuit used to limit the bandwidth of a signal

FLOPPY DISK   A storage medium for digital data after computer processing. Data is stored on a magnetic disk which is protected by a square-shaped flexible cover. Currently, there are two types of floppy disk: 5¼ inch floppy disks and the more sturdy, rigid 3½ inch disks. It is possible to store up to 1.4 megabytes of data on each floppy disk

FM   Frequency modulation: a technique of encoding signals for transmission or recording by causing them to vary a carrier frequency

FRAME   A single television image made up of two interleaved fields

FREQUENCY BAND   Any specified range of frequencies e.g. audio frequency or radio-frequency band

FREQUENCY RESPONSE   The variation in output of a particular component or system across a specified range of frequencies

GAIN   The ratio of output to input signal amplitude or power for an amplifying device or system

GIGA   Prefix, a thousand million times

GLASS ELECTRODE   An electro-chemical electrode whose EMF is pH dependent

HARD DISK   A storage medium for digital data after computer processing which is usually an integral part of the computer system. It is possible to store many hundreds of megabytes of data on each hard disk. It is also common to store computer software for specific applications on the hard disk

HARMONICS   Harmonics are the whole-number multiples of a base frequency known as the fundamental

HARMONIC DISTORTION   The addition of unwanted harmonics to a signal

HERTZ (Hz)   Unit of frequency of vibration. 1 Hz = 1 cycle per second

HIS   Hospital information system

ICU   Intensive Care Unit

IEC   International electrotechnical commission

IMPEDANCE   A measure of the electrical resistance (combined with reactance where this is present) of the input and output of a component or system

ION SENSITIVE ELECTRODE   Electrochemical electrode whose EMF is proportional to the concentration of a particular ion in the medium in which it is immersed e.g. hydrogen, sodium, potassium

ITU   Intensive Therapy Unit

JOULE   Unit of energy

KILO   Prefix, one thousand times

LAN   Local area network. Connects a group of patient monitors or computers and peripheral devices

LCD   Liquid crystal display. Low power consumption, low brightness display utilizing reflected ambient light (usually of digital information)

LED   Light emitting diode. Red LEDs are often used to form bright digital displays

LINEAR   A linear device gives rise to an output signal which exactly mirrors the input over a specified operating range and is free from distortion

LOG IN   The act which establishes a user session on a computer

LUMINANCE   The brightness of a scene

LUX   Unit of illumination

MEGA   Prefix, one million times

MICRO   Prefix, one millionth

MICROPROCESSOR   This is the 'brain' of any computer-based system. Typically, the performance of the microprocessor is measured in terms of its speed of operation, hence 286-, 386-, 486- prefixes, where speed has altered from 8 megahertz to the order of 50 megahertz

MODEM   Modulation/demodulation unit. A device which converts the binary signals of user equipment into audio analogue signals for transmission on a telephone network.

NANO   Prefix, one thousandth of a millionth

NANOMETRE   Unit of optical wavelength

NEWTON   Absolute unit of force

NEWTON PER SQUARE METRE   Absolute unit of pressure also known as the Pascal

NI-CAD   Nickel cadmium. The most popular combination of materials used in portable rechargeable batteries

NOISE   Random unwanted low-level signals

NTC RESISTOR   Negative temperature coefficient resistor (thermistor)

OCTAVE   Span of frequency which represents a doubling or halving of frequency

OHM   Unit of electrical resistance or impedance

OPEN LOOP CONTROL   A control system in which decisions are taken by the clinical user, on the basis of available data pertinent to the patient

OPERATING SYSTEM   Software which controls the execution of computer programs

OPTICAL DISK   A storage medium for digital data after computer processing. It is possible to store many thousands of megabytes of data on each optical disk. It is also the basis of CD-ROM technology from which it is possible to store and retrieve data, but editing of the data is not possible

OR   Operating room

OXIMETER   Device for measuring percentage oxygen saturation

PACS   Picture archiving and communication system

PARTIAL PRESSURE   The % of the total pressure of a gas mixture corresponding with the % by volume of the particular component gas

PASCAL   Absolute unit of pressure, measured in newtons per square metre (Nm^{-2})

% OXYGEN SATURATION   The percentage saturation with oxygen of haemoglobin in blood

PICO   Prefix, one millionth of a millionth

PIN   Personal identification number. A multi-digit code used to confirm and authenticate the identity of a user of a computer-based system

RANDOM ACCESS   The capability to obtain data from a storage device so that the process depends only on the location of the data and not on a reference to data previously accessed

RAM   Random access memory. A memory device which allows direct access for reading or writing to any memory location

REFERENCE ELECTRODE   Provides a stable EMF against which the variable potential from an ion sensitive electrode can be compared

RF   Radio frequency

ROI   Region of interest

SCBU   Special care baby unit

SICU   Surgical intensive care unit

SIGNAL-TO-NOISE RATIO   The ratio of the maximum level of a wanted signal and the background noise remaining when the signal is removed

S-VHS   Super VHS is partly VHS compatible using top quality videotape and component video processing to yield a better-than-broadcast television picture quality for use with X-ray fluoroscopy

TENSION   The equilibrium partial pressure of a component of a gas mixture dissolved in a specified fluid e.g. the tension of carbon dioxide in whole blood might be 13.3 kilopascals

THERMISTOR   Thermally sensitive resistor. Much used in electronic probes to measure body temperature

TONOMETRY   The science of measuring pressure, for example, blood pressure

TRANSDUCER   A device which transduces (transforms) one physical quantity into another e.g. a blood pressure into a corresponding electrical signal

TRANSIENT   A signal of very short duration

ULTRASONIC   Frequencies above the limit of human audibility (i.e. 20 kHz)

VCR   Video cassette recorder

VDU   Visual display unit: another name for the monitor element of a computer system

VHS   Video home system. The Japan Victor Corporation (JVC) originated VCR format which has become the world standard for video cassettes

WORKSTATION   An integrated computer console that offers processing, storage, input and output facilities

Introduction

1

1.1 The high dependency environment

Seriously ill patients can be very dependent for their survival on the provision of a highly supportive environment encompassing both staff and equipment. The high dependency environment obtaining in a hospital is typified by an operating room in which major surgery is performed, or an intensive care unit which can be described as specialized, and confined areas where critically ill patients are gathered together to concentrate both staff expertise and life-support/monitoring equipment. High dependency situations with a more limited time scale occur at the scenes of major accidents and during the transport of the victims to hospital. The creation of such an environment has various consequences. For instance: the highly trained and experienced nurses required to staff the unit can be employed in an efficient and efficacious manner; the sophisticated instrumentation systems needed to enhance patient care are connected to patients for a higher proportion of their operational lifetime. It represents an ideal setting for clinical training of medical, nursing and paramedical staff and for research activities. Such factors contribute to the finding that the presence of a well-staffed and equipped intensive care unit reduces the overall mortality and morbidity of the patients concerned.

Care of the critically ill patient is a phenomenon of the latter half of the twentieth century: the advent of the Second World War acted as a catalyst for the development of patient-management strategies. Owing to the number of casualties involved, specialized approaches were needed to deal with the management of the battle-wounded. For example, in the North African desert campaign of 1943, a thoracic surgical tent was established which dealt only with chest injuries. This enabled the limited number of specialized medical personnel available to be utilized in the most efficient manner.

The management of civilian crises has also been responsible for changes in the care of the critically ill. Indeed, it was the poliomyelitis epidemic of 1952 in Scandinavia which ultimately provided the impetus for the creation of purpose-designed high dependency environments and the development of automatic lung respirators and ventilators. In 1952 no intensive care units existed and in Copenhagen a hospital ward was temporarily adapted to cater for victims of poliomyelitis who suffered from severe respiratory problems caused by their primary illness.

This ward was supervized by anaesthetists and the treatment regimes in use were described by Ibsen, B. (1954) 'The anaesthetist's viewpoint on treatment of respiratory complications in poliomyelitis during the epidemic in Copenhagen, 1952', *Proceedings of the Royal Society of Medicine*, **47**, 52. As the available technology had yet to improve on the performance of the Cuirass respirator, intermittent positive pressure ventilation was applied manually to the tracheostomized patients by 'bag squeezing' for prolonged periods of time, using volunteers.

Clinical acceptance of this regime of treatment was enhanced because it could be evaluated objectively: Lassen, H. C. A. (1953) 'Preliminary report of the 1952 epidemic of poliomyelitis in Copenhagen. With special reference to the treatment of acute respiratory insufficiency' The *Lancet*, **1**, 37. Epidemiologists could compare the mortality rates from respiratory paralysis occurring during the poliomyelitis outbreak with those from a similar outbreak in Scandinavia which had occurred three years previously. The results were conclusive: throughout Scandinavia the mortality rate during the 1949 epidemic was 85%. Before the intervention by anaesthetists in the Danish 1952 epidemic, the mortality rate was 87%. After therapeutic intervention as described above, the mortality rate decreased by more than one half i.e. to 40%.

The clinical knowledge gained from these experiences had at least two significant consequences. First, a technological advance was achieved in the design of automatic lung ventilators and the administration of intermittent positive pressure ventilation. Second, a methodological advance occurred with the design of a special unit catering for the care of critically ill patients.

The first purpose-built civilian multi-disciplinary intensive care units opened almost simultaneously in Baltimore, USA, and in Uppsala, Sweden, in 1958. The latter unit illustrates the improvements made in design with 22 beds split into two wards. The larger of the two wards contained 13 beds and was in the charge of anaesthetists; this could be considered as an extension of the post-operative recovery room. It developed into the medico-surgical intensive care unit. The second ward of nine beds was in the charge of cardio-thoracic surgeons and represents, perhaps, the original coronary care unit.

Other specialist units which can be considered under the category of high dependency environments exhibit a more chequered development, owing much to the personality of individual clinicians rather than to any structured advance in methodology for patient care. Harvey, A. M. (1974) 'Neurosurgical genius – Walter Edward Dandy', *John Hopkins Medical Journal*, **135**, 358–68 describes one such individual. Walter Dandy was responsible for establishing a three-bed neurosurgical intensive care unit in Baltimore in 1923.

A neonatal intensive care unit was in existence in Chicago in 1927. However, the treatment regimes were still very crude, often using medical instrumentation designed for adults on neonates because there was no alternative. However, the availability of the unit encouraged the construction of purpose-built equipment.

A joint report by the Royal College of Surgeons of England and the British Association of Paediatric Surgeons (October 1992) on 'Surgical Services for the Newborn' states that the efficient function of a neonatal surgical intensive care unit requires the services of paediatric anaesthesia, nurses trained in the care of the newborn, paediatricians with experience of neonatology, paediatric radiology and ultrasonography, biochemical services with micromethods, paediatric pathology and microbiology, paediatric oncology and cytology and clinical geneticists.

A minimum of 12 neonatal cots should be available with up to 6 staffed for intensive care and the remainder staffed for high dependency and special care. Suitable nurse to patient ratios are: for intensive care 5.5:1; for high dependency 3:1 and for special care 1.5:1. For a unit of 12 cots this equates to a total of 51 ($6 \times 5.5 + 6 \times 3$) whole-time equivalent nurses of whom at least 70% should be registered sick children's trained nurses, the remaining 30% can be registered general or enrolled nurses (general).

With the establishment of high dependency environments within a hospital, the emphasis has now changed from the development of clinical life-support techniques to the evolution of appropriate technology. The use of on-line computers for the continuous monitoring of physiological signals became practicable in 1964 in Los Angeles. The availability of new technologies has been manifested in the advances seen with automatic lung ventilators, blood-gas analysers and pulse oximeters. As but one example, a blood sample volume of only 40 microlitres is capable of providing a reliable blood-gas reading for a neonate. Thus, serial determinations are feasible with even the smallest baby.

1.2 Technology applied to intensive care

It is the purpose of clinical measurement to provide data, which on interpretation yields information concerning the physiological well-being of the patient. Such measurements can be classified in many ways, one of the most simple being the distinction between on-line and off-line data. On-line data might originate continuously from a blood pressure transducer and off-line data be logged manually as with a body-temperature thermometer or the collection bottle connected to a urethral catheter.

'Intelligent' instrumentation based on the power of microcomputers renders possible the much more stringent and rapid calibration and data-validity checks required in order to be able to handle large amounts of on-line information with confidence. A well-thought-out patient-monitoring system can relieve doctors and nurses of much routine checking of data but even so, human vigilance and commonsense is still essential. Classification is also possible in terms of the measurement technique employed. For example, the term 'laboratory data' can be used to describe those measurements made on biological samples in areas such as the chemical pathology, haematology and microbiology laboratories.

It is also possible to devise a classification system which compounds some of these terms, e.g. 'discrete monitored data' and 'continuous monitored data' could be admissible categories. An example of a classification system with a particular measurement in each category is:

- discrete laboratory data – serum electrolytes
- discrete monitored data – non-invasive blood pressure
- continuous monitored data – electrocardiogram
- 'other' patient data – age, height, weight

These are direct measurements or observations. It is also possible to use derived measurements. Here several direct measurements are employed in conjunction with one another to yield additional (sometimes more informative) patient data. For example, normalization of data allows comparisons to be made between patients. The cardiac index takes into account the size of the patient. The cardiac index is given by the cardiac output divided by the body-surface area of the patient and is expressed in litres per minute per square metre. The surface area is usually calculated by means of a nomogram based on the patient's height and weight.

A complete system of measurement will include the patient, the sensor, the associated instrumentation system and the observer. It is important to remember that the true (absolute) value of the variable is not necessarily identical with the measured value because of the presence of errors in the measurement arrangement, Figure 1.1. Measurement has an essential role to play in high dependency environments as it provides quantitative data concerning the condition of the patients. The wide range of measurements now feasible require an equally wide range of instrumentation systems.

Figure 1.1 The effect of error causing the measured value to differ from the true value of a variable.

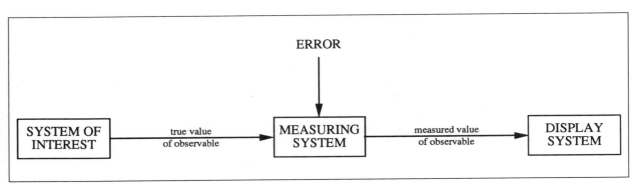

Figure 1.2 illustrates the wide range of physiological data which is usually required and which is collected, processed and displayed with equipment such as that shown in Figure 1.3. Sensors or transducers are needed which can respond to changes in physiological pressures, flows, volumes, temperatures, bioelectric signals and biochemical processes. Some of the sensors, such as those responding to respiratory gas flows, may be in direct contact with the measured variable. Others make an indirect contact. For example, in the measurement of arterial blood pressure, a saline filled cannula is often interposed between the site of measurement (perhaps in the brachial artery) and the transducer which is

PRESSURES
    Arterial blood pressure   (systolic, diastolic)
    Venous blood pressure
    Pulmonary capillary wedge pressure
    Intra-cranial pressure

FLOWS
    Blood flow
    Respiratory gas flow

VOLUMES
    Tidal volume
    Minute volume

TEMPERATURE
    Core temperature
    Peripheral temperature (big toe)

INPUTS
    Drugs and their doses

OUTPUTS
    Cardiac output

INPUT–OUTPUT RELATIONSHIP
    Fluid-electrolyte balance

ELECTROPHYSIOLOGICAL SIGNALS
    Electrocardiogram
    Electroencephalogram
    Evoked responses

BIOCHEMISTRY
    Electrolytes
    Liver function tests

Figure 1.2 A wide range of physiological variables which can be encountered in intensive care situations.

external to the patient. The pulsatile nature of the arterial pressure can often be observed in terms of the oscillations of the blood-saline interface. It is the change in pressure of the saline acting on the diaphragm of the transducer which is recorded as a proxy for the true blood pressure. The recorded pressure waveform is dependent upon factors such as the presence of a compressible air bubble and the rigidity of the walls of the cannula and its length as well as the characteristics of the transducer.

A more abstract measurement process arises in the recording of data due to electrophysiological activity. Here, the transmission of the signal in the body via ionic currents in tissue must be converted to an electronic

Figure 1.3 Patient monitoring system. (By courtesy of Hewlett-Packard Ltd.)

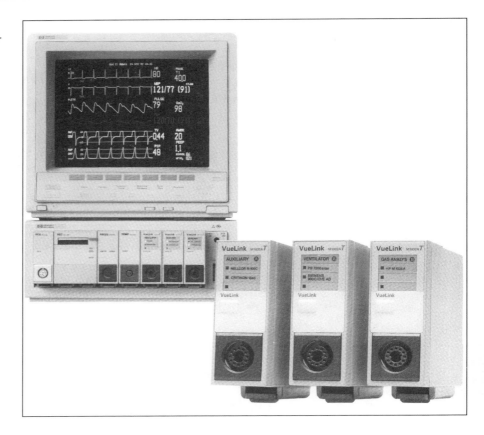

current which is collected by appropriate electrodes. This conversion occurs at the patient-electrode interface. The electrophysiological signal detected at the electrodes may already be weakened, especially if the activity to be recorded arises from structures deep within the body or is screened by the skull, as occurs with the electroencephalogram (EEG).

The role of measurement in the planning of therapy is clear: the more firm data that can be collected, recorded and displayed via the wide range of instrumentation systems found at the patient's bedside and beyond, the greater is the information available to the clinical design-maker. On this basis, the most appropriate treatment can be prescribed for the well-being of the patient. Thus it is crucial that an understanding of the principles of clinical measurement and medical instrumentation is acquired by nurses working in intensive care situations, since they act as the pivot for providing care for the majority of the time spent by a patient in hospital.

Nurses working in a high dependency environment are likely to be busy, concentrating on the responsibilities of their duties and often under stress. Hence it is important that any equipment used should be easy to set up, provided with a clear set of operating instructions and that the data/information produced should be readily visible and interpretable. At all times, technology should be employed to enhance the care of patients by skilled staff and not simply as a substitute for staff.

Underpinning knowledge of physics and computing

2

In order to be able to understand the operator's manuals and obtain a knowledge of the operating principles of medical devices encountered in their work, it is necessary for nurses to acquire an understanding of certain concepts and definitions used in areas such as electrical science, mechanics and optics.

The use of personal computers and the microprocessors on which they are based is becoming commonplace in the clinical environment. They can be found in the form of 'stand-alone' devices, for example, a dedicated computer system used for a specific purpose such as the calculation of drug dosage or fluid balance requirements in a burns unit. Alternatively, they can be integrated into medical equipment to the extent that the end-user can remain in ignorance of their presence. For example, the Puritan Bennett Model 7200A ventilator is controlled by a microprocessor which is crucial to the functioning of the ventilator. To the uninitiated, computing terminology can be considered as a jungle of jargon. However, it is becoming increasingly important for nurses to understand the key concepts involved in computing, as computers affect more of their working lives. In this book, computing terms are introduced in such a fashion as to dispel some of the myths which can surround their use.

This background will make for an easier relationship with the equipment and also with the manufacturer's representatives and those responsible for maintenance and repairs.

2.1 Electrical science

2.1.1 Types of electricity

2.1.1.1 Static electricity

As the name implies, static electricity consists of stationary charges of electricity and these are resident on an insulated surface. Static electric charges usually result from friction between two such surfaces which subsequently rapidly become separated. Rubbing a glass rod with a dry cloth and then rapidly separating the rod and cloth is an example.

The charged object can discharge if it comes close to an earthed object producing a spark. Thus a person wearing rubber-soled shoes and walking across man-made fibre carpeting in a modern hotel can experience a small shock when touching a lift-call button which discharges the charge accumulated on the person. High voltages can be generated in this way but very little current is available. However, the energy liberated can be sufficient to produce a microspark capable of igniting an explosive mixture of ether and oxygen to cause a lethal explosion in an operating room unless anti-static precautions have been observed. These include the provision of a conducting terrazzo floor, spark-proof equipment, anti-static rubber and cotton outer garments for staff. These are no longer required in operating and anaesthetic rooms unless flammable anaesthetic agents such as ether and cyclopropane are in use.

However, a build-up of static charge can cause unwanted sudden deflections on the screen of ECG monitors and unwanted shocks when staff wearing man-made fibre clothes touch each other. These problems can be minimized by using anti-static rubber tubing and trolley-wheel tyres to prevent the build-up of high voltage static charges. Plastic articles can be sprayed with a conducting spray to leak away charges.

2.1.1.2 Current electricity

Direct current (d.c.) electricity consists of electric charges flowing in one direction only in a conducting pathway or circuit such as a wire. It is produced by a rotating electrical machine – a dynamo – or more usually by a battery in the case of portable devices such as ambulatory patient monitors and vehicle batteries used for powering equipment in ambulances.

Low voltage d.c. supplies are commonly encountered in powering motors to move the patient couch of an X-ray system or lamps forming part of an optical device. Although the voltage involved may be no more than 12 volts, considerable current may be available and under fault conditions involving metal electrodes placed on the skin a patient can suffer a nasty electrolytic burn beneath an electrode which has become connected to a d.c. voltage. The passage of the current drives metal ions into the skin. Alternating current (a.c.) supplies pass the current alternately in a forward and then in a reverse direction around the circuit. The number of times per second the current flows in either the forward or the reverse direction is known as the frequency of the a.c. supply. The usual mains electricity supply in British and European hospitals is 50 cycles per second, whereas in North America it is 60 cycles per second. Each cycle includes one forward and one reverse flow of current. One cycle per second is called one Hertz (Hz). One thousand hertz is one kilohertz (kHz) and one million hertz is one megahertz (MHz).

Figure 2.1 illustrates the waveform of a 50 Hz 240 volt root mean square (r.m.s.) mains voltage, typical of that encountered in the United Kingdom.

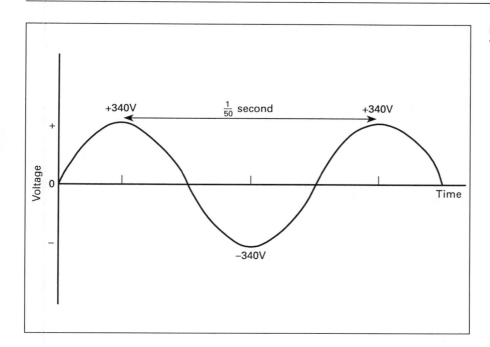

Figure 2.1 Waveform of a 240 volt r.m.s. 50 Hz mains supply.

The waveform is sinusoidal and consists of an alternate series of positive and negative peaks, each complete cycle occupying one fiftieth (20 milliseconds) of a second. The peak values are plus or minus 340 volts and the insulation of wiring used with this mains voltage must be designed to withstand the peak voltages.

The usual mains supply for equipment used in intensive care situations is a single phase a.c. supply provided via two cores of a 3-core mains cable. These are the line and neutral leads. The third core is the earth lead. This is connected directly to earth and is at a potential of zero volts. The neutral lead will normally be at a potential close to earth, while the line lead for a 240 volt r.m.s. a.c. supply will alternate between plus and minus 340 volts.

In the United Kingdom the insulation of the line lead of a mains cable is coloured brown, the neutral blue and the earth yellow and green stripes. The earth lead must be sufficiently substantial that it can carry a short circuit current from the line lead to earth. It is connected to the largest pin of a 3-pin mains plug. The line lead connects to this pin via a suitable cartridge fuse, typical fuse ratings being 2, 5 and 13 amperes. If the fuse rating is too small, blown fuses may arise due to an initial current surge arising when equipment is first switched on. Special 'slow blow' fuses are fitted to some electronic equipment and are rated to pass the surge current. The line and neutral leads should not be interchanged when a plug is fitted to a mains cable. Mains cables, and indeed other external cables connected to equipment, are vulnerable to mechanical damage or straining, for example, if they are run over by a trolley, or the equipment trolley is pulled away from the wall in which the mains outlet is located. The cable insulation can be cut or the earth lead pulled away from its pin in the mains plug. Each time equipment is plugged into the mains, a quick visible inspection of the cable for integrity and the plug for loose connections is a simple procedure which pays dividends.

The human heart is particularly at risk from shock involving mains frequency supplies, whereas higher frequencies, typically in the range 20 kHz to 100 kHz, pose a negligible hazard to the heart and are commonly used in devices such as impedance pneumographs for monitoring the respiratory rate. Zero frequency is often referred to as d.c. since a direct current is continuous and exhibits no alternations of direction. Frequencies of up to a few tens of thousands of hertz are loosely grouped as audio frequencies; frequencies higher than this are known as radio frequencies. As an example, the BBC 1500 metre long-wave radio station at Rugby operates on a frequency of 200 kHz. Surgical diathermy sets produce radio frequency power in the frequency range 0.5 to 1.5 MHz. Localized heating of breast tumours (hyperthermia) is performed with microwaves in the frequency range 800 to 1000 MHz.

Mains, audio and radio frequency electricity supplies are examples of electromagnetic radiations. They travel at the speed of light, 300 million metres per second. The number of waves (cycles) occurring per second is the frequency. Dividing the velocity by the frequency gives the distance travelled in one cycle which is the wavelength. Thus velocity (metres per second) = wavelength (in metres) $\times$ frequency (in Hz). It is worth noting that diagnostic ultrasound scanners (often used in coronary care and obstetric units) emit beams of ultrasound (sound with a frequency higher than the audible range) with frequencies typically in the range 3 to 7 MHz. However, sound and ultrasound consists of trains of pressure pulses which can only travel through a medium such as air, water or tissue in contrast to electromagnetic waves which can travel through a vacuum such as outer space.

The fact that radio frequencies can penetrate tissue allows a radio link from a hand-held control box containing a small transmitter and aerial to feed electrical power and control signals to the receiving aerial of an electronic implant beneath the patient's skin, such as a stimulator for pain relief or a cardiac pacemaker, without the need for a direct electrical connection. A beam of ultrasound will also penetrate tissue but is subject to reflection at tissue-fluid interfaces and this fact complicates the interpretation of medical ultrasound images obtained by scanning the volume of tissue of interest with a beam of ultrasound and viewing the reflected signals in an appropriate way to form the image required.

2.1.2 Fundamentals and harmonics

The simplest alternating current waveform, typically that of the a.c. mains supply, is sinusoidal. This waveform would appear across the ends of a coil of wire which was rotated at a steady speed in the magnetic field existing between the pole pieces of a permanent magnet forming a simple alternator for generating alternating current. If the coil makes 50 complete rotations in one second, the frequency of the current generated is 50 Hz. In practice, electrophysiological waveforms, such as that of the arterial blood pressure, are more complex. The waveform can be shown to consist of a series of frequency-related components of varying amplitudes. Essentially it comprises a fundamental frequency sinewave plus a number of harmonically related sinewaves which may have frequencies of double, treble and higher multiples of the fundamental. The output waveform of a spark-gap surgical-diathermy set comprises a sinewave at the fundamental frequency plus a large number of harmonic components. In a given waveform not all of the even and odd harmonics may be present.

A heart rate of 60 beats per minute has a fundamental frequency of 1 Hz. For a faithful reproduction of the arterial waveform a recording channel should have a frequency response which is linear out to at least the 10th harmonic and for the reproduction of small notches the bandwidth should extend out to the 20th harmonic.

2.1.3 Units of electric current

The unit of electric current is the ampere. A compact ECG and heart-rate monitor might draw two amperes from a 12 volt car battery when used in an ambulance. This is direct current. In the case of alternating current the ampere is still used as the unit of current but it now refers to the equivalent a.c. current which would produce the same heating power. Electric current gives rise to heat as it flows through a circuit. If the current was one ampere d.c. the equivalent for a.c. is one ampere root mean square (r.m.s.). For the compact monitor, if it was powered from a 240 volt a.c. mains supply, the current drawn from the mains would amount to 0.1 amperes r.m.s. at 50 Hz since in each case the power consumption is 24 watts (see section 2.1.7).

In a simple circuit comprising resistors only, the voltage and current waveforms will be sinusoidal and in step (in phase). Suppose that the circuit resistance amounted to 50 ohms and the mains voltage applied across it was 240 volts r.m.s. By Ohm's Law the current flowing is 240/50 = 4.8 amperes r.m.s. The heating power in watts dissipated in the circuit is 240 × 4.8 = 1152 watts = 1.152 kilowatts. The same heating power would be developed if a d.c. voltage of 240 was applied across the circuit. The peak voltages are plus and minus 340 volts and the peak currents are 6.8 amperes in the forward and reverse directions. It is important that the type of resistor chosen should be able to dissipate the power developed in it without overheating or burning adjacent components or a patient.

Currents of a few milliamperes r.m.s. (1000 milliamperes = 1 ampere) at a frequency of about 100 kHz would flow through a patient's thorax during electrical impedance monitoring of his cardiac output, while currents of 100 microamperes (1 million microamperes = 1 ampere) at a mains frequency of 50 Hz might interfere with the pumping action of the heart.

2.1.4 Units of electric voltage

A source of electrical pressure (voltage) in the form of a battery, electronic power supply or a mains supply is required to drive electric current through the resistance of a circuit. The unit of voltage is the volt. A set of three 1.5 volt batteries can power a portable tape recorder used for dictation. One kilovolt is equal to 1000V and voltages of several kilovolts are encountered in defibrillators. Voltages of several million volts (megavolts) are encountered with devices generating beams of powerful X-rays for use in radiotherapy.

One millivolt is one thousandth of a volt and the R-wave of an normal ECG would have an amplitude of approximately one to two millivolts. One microvolt is one millionth of a volt and the amplitude of an electroencephalogram (EEG) from the brain might be about 100 microvolts when recorded from electrodes located on the scalp.

2.1.5 Units of electrical resistance

Electric current flows in a circuit under the influence of a voltage applied across the circuit. The opposition to current flow, strictly speaking in the case of a direct current, is expressed in terms of the circuit resistance. This is measured in ohms. A voltage of one volt applied across a circuit of one ohm resistance will give rise to a current of one ampere. The resistance of the heart is approximately 50 ohms and the skin-contact resistance of an ECG electrode assuming a good skin preparation and a firm contact is a few thousand ohms. In a simple resistive circuit Ohm's Law states that the application of a voltage V to a circuit of resistance R ohms gives rise to a current of V/R amperes.

2.1.6 Unit of electrical and other forms of energy

Electricity is just one form of energy. Electrical energy can be converted to alternative forms e.g. into heat energy in a radiant heater used in the resuscitation of infants or into sound energy via a headphone or loudspeaker. The unit of energy is the joule. A typical defibrillator discharge might amount to 200 joules. Energy is the capacity for doing work. In defibrillation the 'stored work' from the charged capacitor is expended with the intention of restoring the fibrillating heart to a sinus rhythm. The requirement to quantify available energy also occurs in nutrition. The energy provided per gram of nutrient expressed in kilojoules (1000 J) is 17 for protein, 37 for fat and 16 for carbohydrate (expressed as monosaccharide). A knowledge of the energy available is particularly important when the patient is dependent upon parenteral nutrition. As an example, premature infants require an energy intake per day in the range 420 to 530 kilojoules.

2.1.7 Unit of electrical and other forms of power

Power is the rate of doing work. The unit is the watt and is familiar in the form of the power rating of electric lamps e.g. a 100 watt bulb. The power consumption of a portable patient monitor for ECG, pulse rate and body temperature is quoted as 40 watts and it can be powered from the a.c. mains, a sealed rechargeable lead-acid battery pack or external-vehicle battery supply in the range 11 to 22 volts d.c.. If an electrically powered item of equipment draws A amperes of current from a supply of V volts, the power consumed is the product (V × A) watts. A German make of electronically controlled automatic lung ventilator is quoted as drawing 0.75 amperes at the continental supply voltage of 220V. The power used is 165 watts. A surgical diathermy unit might be capable of producing a maximum radio frequency power output of 400 watts.

The unit of electrical power consumption is the kilowatt hour and this is the unit for which electricity power-supply companies quote a charge in terms of the energy supplied. A one kilowatt electric fire burning for one hour consumes one unit of electricity. The ventilator previously quoted as drawing 0.75 amperes from a 220 volt supply consumes 0.165 units of electricity per hour. Since there are 60 × 60 = 3600 seconds in one hour and 1 kilowatt = 1000 watts, one kilowatt is the same as 3 600 000 joules i.e. 3.6 MJ.

The watt is also used as a unit of optical power e.g. a 100 watt carbon dioxide surgical laser and also as a measure of heat loss in patients. The various forms of heat loss occurring in a one-day-old 0.75 kg premature baby at 27 weeks gestation in still air at 36 degrees Celsius have been given as approximately 2 watts per square metre due to radiation, 13 watts per square metre due to evaporation and 2 watts per square metre due to convection. As another example, an alarm will sound with some types of infra-red radiant warmer used in the resuscitation of neonates when the radiant heat emission falling on the baby exceeds a level of 10 milliwatts per square centimetre where 1000 milliwatts = 1 watt.

2.2 Mechanics

2.2.1 System of units

Mechanics may be defined as the subject in which the conditions under which objects around us move or are at rest are studied. A system of units for use in subject areas related to mechanics is based upon specifying convenient units for mass, length and time. The system now universally used in Europe for scientific applications is the SI system (Systeme Internationale d'Unites). The SI system is based upon multiples of ten, each unit being expressed as multiples or sub-multiples. Thus: mega (one million), kilo (one thousand), hecto (one hundred), deca (ten), deci (one tenth), centi (one hundredth), milli (one thousandth), micro (one millionth), nano (one thousandth of a millionth), pico (one millionth of a millionth).

2.2.2 Unit of mass

Mass is defined as the quantity of matter in a body and the unit of mass on the SI system is the kilogram. Weight is the term used for the force due to gravity acting on a body which causes it to fall towards earth when dropped. Thus the force due to gravity acting on a man of mass 70 kg is 70 kg weight and it is this force which is measured when the ward scales are used to weigh a patient.

2.2.3 Dimensional units

The SI system unit of length is the metre. e.g. a patient's height of 1.5 metres. His body surface area will be expressed in square metres i.e. 1.89 square metres using the Dubois formula (DuBois, D. and Dubois, E. F. (1916) 'A formula to estimate the approximate surface area if height and weight be known', *Archives of Internal Medicine*, **16** 863). If his cardiac output was 4.8 litres per minute his cardiac index is 2.54 litres per minute per square metre. However, if his mass was 70 kg, his body mass index is $70/(1.5 \times 1.5) = 31.1$ kg per metre squared. Values in excess of 40 may be considered as appropriate to an obese patient.

2.2.4 Unit of time

The SI system unit of time is the second, but minutes and hours are used for the longer periods of time. The millisecond (1/1000 second) is used for measurements of the cardiac cycle e.g. a left ventricular ejection time (LVET) of 350 ms. LVET is defined as the time interval between the systolic upstroke of the arterial blood pressure waveform and the incisura of the dicrotic notch.

The total electromechanical time of the cardiac contraction is taken as the time interval between the onset of the QRS complex of the ECG and the first fast component of the second heart sound of the phonocardiogram. This is the Q-S2 interval. The pre-ejection period (PEP) is taken as the difference between (Q-S2) and LVET. The PEP/LVET ratio has been used as an index of the state of the heart's myocardial contractility. Possible values might be LVET = 350 ms, PEP = 100 ms, PEP/LVET = 0.29.

2.2.5 Unit of velocity

Velocity is the distance travelled (strictly in a specified direction) per unit time so that on the SI system the unit of velocity is the metre per second. The peak ejection velocity of blood expelled from a patient's left ventricle might be one metre per second.

2.2.6 Unit of volume flow

The product of the velocity of the fluid involved multiplied by the cross-sectional area of the vessel concerned gives the volume flow in litres per minute. If a patient's aorta has a diameter of 1.5 cm, the cross-sectional area is 1.75 square centimetres and for a peak ejection velocity of one metre per second the peak blood volume flow is 0.175 litres per second or 10.2 litres per minute.

A knowledge of volume flow rates is important when setting up infusion devices. For example, a volumetric infusion pump used in a special care baby unit for dextrose and total parenteral-nutrition infusions with neonates of body weight 0.95 kg to 3 kg can be set with incremental volume flow rates of 0.1 ml per hour over the range 0.1 to 99.9 ml per hour.

2.2.7 Unit of acceleration

Acceleration is defined as rate of change of velocity. An object which is dropped and falls freely towards the earth's surface attains an acceleration due to the force of gravity acting on it of 9.8 metres per second per second i.e. the object's velocity increases by 9.8 metres per second for each second of travel. Acceleration is associated with an increase of velocity while deceleration implies a decreasing velocity. Rapid deceleration as in car crashes can produce serious trauma to the human body.

2.2.8 Unit of force

The application of force is required to accelerate a body and the SI unit of force is the newton. It is independent of gravity and is that force which will give a mass of 1 kg an acceleration of one metre per second per second. The force required to move a particular item of equipment may be detailed in a specification e.g. to move a ceiling-suspended X-ray tube mount should not require a force in excess of 50 newtons.

2.2.9 Units of pressure

Pressure is defined as force per unit area. The SI unit of pressure is the pascal which is equal to one newton per square metre. Blood-gas tensions are commonly quoted in kilopascals e.g. a PO_2 of 13 kPa and a PCO_2 of 5.2 kPa where one kilopascal equals 1000 pascals. Medical gas cylinder and pipeline pressures are also quoted in kilopascals. Thus an oxygen cylinder pressure gauge would be scaled from 0 to 300 kilopascals. Hospital vacuum pipeline gauges are scaled from 0 to 30 kilopascals or 0 to 100 kilopascals in an anti-clockwise direction depending on whether they are intended for low or high suction applications.

Historically, physiological pressures have been quoted in terms of the height of the column of a specified fluid which the pressure could support (as in a mercury barometer for measuring atmospheric pressure). Thus blood pressure is commonly quoted in terms of millimetres of mercury, although central venous pressures may be quoted in terms of centimetres of water (in practice, sterile saline). It is worth remembering that 1 cm of mercury is equivalent to 13.6 cm of water and 1 mm Hg = 133 pascals. In North America blood-gas tensions can be given in torr (Torricelli). This is a non-SI unit and 1 torr = 1 mm of mercury. A standard atmosphere is taken as 760 mm of mercury and one atmosphere is also equivalent to a pressure of 14.7 pounds weight per square inch (psi). The pound per square inch is an engineering unit of pressure widely used in the past in hospital engineering circles for gas-cylinder and pipeline (60 psi) pressures.

2.3 Logarithms

When dealing with very large or very small numbers or wide ranges of a particular quantity the calculations are made more convenient to handle by arranging to work in terms of indices. As an example, one million equals 10 multiplied by itself 6 times i.e. 10 raised to the power 6 and one millionth equals 10 raised to the power minus 6. The power to which a fixed number (the base) must be raised to produce a given number is called the logarithm of that number to that particular base. Index notation is commonly encountered e.g. a range of light intensities of 10 000 to 1 becomes 10^4 to 1.

Thus, 6 is the logarithm to the base 10 of one million and 2 is the logarithm to the base 10 of 100. Logarithms to the base 10 are called common logarithms. Natural logarithms are to a base of 2.71828. This value 2.71828 is known as the exponential (e). Power series consisting of a number of terms each having 'e' raised to a different power are commonly encountered. A relevant example occurs with the Dundee five-year risk factor for coronary heart disease: Tunstall-Pedoe, H. (1991) 'The Dundee coronary-risk disk for management of change in risk factors', *British Medical Journal*, **303**, 744–7.

The formula for the five-year risk is $1/(1 + e$ to the power $-(a + b_1X_1 + b_2X_2 + b_3X_3 + b_4X_4)$ where $a = -10.117$ and is a constant, $b_1 = 0.0651$, $X_1 =$ the patient's age in years, $b_2 = 0.01054$, $X_2 =$ the patient's systolic blood pressure in mmHg, $b_3 = 0.3627$, $X_3 =$ the patient's cholesterol level in mmol per litre, $b_4 = 1$ and X_4 is a smoking code (0 for non-smoker, 0.4483 for 1–9 cigarettes per day; 0.9242 for 10; 1.1019 for 11 to 19; 0.9333 for 20; 1.236 for 21–29 and 1.431 for 30 or more cigarettes per day).

Using this formula a 30-year-old man with a systolic blood pressure of 100 mmHg, a cholesterol level of 5 mmol per litre and a non-smoker has a risk factor of 0.005. A 50-year-old man with a systolic blood pressure of 120 mmHg, a cholesterol level of 7 mmol per litre and smoking 20 cigarettes per day has a risk factor of 0.107 which is 21 times greater than the non-smoking 30-year-old, while a 50-year-old man with a systolic pressure of 130 mmHg, a cholesterol level of 8 mmol per litre and smoking more than 30 cigarettes per day now has a risk factor of 0.24: some 48 times greater than for the non-smoking 30-year-old.

On ordinary linear graph paper, equal divisions of the scales for the axes represent equal additions of the quantities concerned, whereas with logarithmic graph paper equal divisions of the scales present equal multiplications of the quantities concerned. The power gain of an audio amplifier is usually adjustable over quite a wide range, perhaps up to a gain of several thousands. The gain can be expressed in terms of decibels (dB) where the gain in dB equals 10 times the common logarithm of (P_{out}/P_{in})

where P_{in} and P_{out} are respectively the input and output powers of the amplifier measured across identical values of resistance.

If the gain of an amplifier is expressed not in terms of the ratio of output to input power but output voltage V_{out} to input voltage V_{in}, the expression for the gain in dB becomes 20 times the common logarithm of (V_{out}/V_{in}). The factor 20 arises from the fact that the power developed in a resistor is proportional to the square of the voltage appearing across it.

The common mode rejection ratio for a Japanese Fukuda Denshi ECG recorder is quoted as better than 100 dB i.e. 100 000 to 1. Its frequency response is quoted as 0.05 Hz to 100 Hz, these being the 3 dB points. In general, the frequency response of an amplifier is fairly flat over quite a wide range of frequencies but will reduce at both the lower and upper limits of the range. It is conventional to define the lower and upper limits of the frequency response in terms of the half-power points. A fall in power of 50% is equivalent to a loss of 3 dB so that the limits of the response are known as the 3 dB points. For the Fukuda Denshi ECG recorder the quoted 3 dB points are 0.05 Hz and 100 Hz. The upper 3 dB point is set by the response of the heated stylus arm of the chart recorder.

The whole concept of pH is based upon the use of logarithms. As a simplification it can be taken that the pH value of a blood sample is equal to –1 multiplied by the power to which 10 must be raised to equal the hydrogen ion concentration of the blood. A pH value of 7 units indicates a hydrogen ion concentration of 10 to the power -7 moles per litre. Blood-gas analysers contain a pH sensitive glass electrode in combination with a reference electrode. A typical blood pH range would be 6.000 to 8.000 pH units.

2.4 Units of light wavelength

Light, like radio waves, is a form of electromagnetic radiation. Visible light which can be perceived by the eye encompasses all the colours of the rainbow from violet at the short wavelength end of the visible spectrum to red at the long wavelength end. Wavelengths which are too short to be visible to the eye fall in the ultraviolet region of the spectrum while those which are too long fall in the infra-red.

The unit of light wavelength is the nanometre (nm) which is 10 to the power –9 metres. Oximeters used for the measurement of the percentage oxygen saturation of haemoglobin operate on two wavelengths, 660 nm in the red and 940 nm in the infra-red. A phototherapy lamp used with jaundiced neonates emits its maximum energy in the intense blue region of the spectrum at 460 nm which is close to the absorption peak of bilirubin. If the therapy results obtained at 460 nm are taken as 100%, light of wavelength 435 and 490 nm would be only half as efficient, while there would be no absorption at wavelengths of 410 or 530 nm.

For wavelengths in the longer wavelength part of the infra-red region the micrometre (1000 nm) is used. Capnography is the measurement of the partial pressure of carbon dioxide in the expired air of a patient. It utilizes the fact that carbon dioxide strongly absorbs at 4.25 micrometres. Nitrous oxide absorbs at 4.49 micrometres. Compact infra-red analysers are often used with anaesthetic machines for the continuous monitoring of the concentrations in the anaesthetic circuit of carbon dioxide, nitrous oxide and volatile agents such as halothane or enflurane.

2.5 Photometric units

The SI unit of light energy collected within a specified beam angle is the lumen which is equivalent to 0.00146 watts. In intensive care units and operating rooms the level of illumination is important in terms of the comfort of patients and of staff performing delicate tasks. The SI unit of intensity of illumination is the lux (one lumen per square metre) and a general level of illumination in operating rooms is 800 to 1000 lux. Fluorescent lamps are commonly employed to produce high intensity shadow-free lighting in high dependency areas of hospitals. The colour rendering of the lamp phosphors must be chosen so as not to inhibit the detection of incipient cyanosis in patients.

2.6 Computer concepts

The key computer concepts which must be understood embrace the terms: hardware; software; storage and communication. Having this information at your fingertips means that some sense can be made of the manuals which accompany computer or microprocessor-based medical instrumentation.

2.6.1 Hardware

The hardware of a computer system can be described basically as those items which you can see and this is shown schematically in Figure 2.2(a). It comprises a keyboard used for manually entering data, a monitor (sometimes called a visual display unit or VDU) for viewing input and output, and the 'black box' part – known as the system unit. In some configurations there may also be a printer – another output device from which hard copy may be obtained which may simply be a print-out of the information displayed on the monitor. The keyboard and monitor, together with a storage device known as a floppy disk (modern disks are not actually floppy but have inherited the name) are shown on the left-hand side of Figure 2.2(a). It is the system unit which contains the electronic 'brain' of the computer, known as the central processing unit (CPU). This is shown on the right-hand side of Figure 2.2(a) together with only some of the elements which also form part of the system unit.

Communication between the system unit and the other elements of the computer system, is achieved by means of specific device controllers (DCs) which are connected to the CPU via the input/output (I/O) control unit.

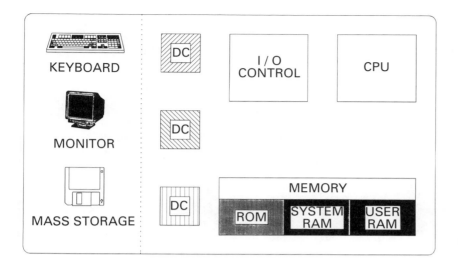

Figure 2.2(a) Computer hardware: schematic view. (Courtesy P. J. Hamilton.)

Whenever a new peripheral is added on to the computer system, it must be accompanied by its own device controller. For instance, a popular way to input data is via a pointing device such as a 'mouse' or trackerball. When these are connected, space must be found within the system unit for all their device controllers, otherwise the system will not function at all.

It is essential for its operation that the computer system 'remembers' data. As indicated in Figure 2.2(a) computer memory is divided into two basic types: read-only memory (ROM) and random access memory (RAM). ROM is also known as memory which is 'hard-wired'. Any computer program stored in ROM is permanent, and is inserted there by the supplier of the computer equipment. It cannot be altered by the user in any way. Hence the term 'read-only'. Computer software may be provided in hard-wired form for legal and ethical reasons so that responsibility for it is unambiguous, as is the case for the Puritan-Bennett Model 7200A ventilator.

In contrast to ROM, RAM is temporary (volatile) in nature, and any computer program stored in RAM will be erased when the computer is switched off – unless the RAM is provided with a short-term power supply such as a battery to provide back-up until the power is restored. RAM is further divided into system RAM and user RAM. The programs which are required before any use can be made of the computer are transferred to RAM from either an external source via a floppy disk, or from an internal source known as a 'hard disk'. Since not all computer systems are provided with a hard disk, it has been omitted from Figure 2.2(a). Figure 2.2(b) shows a typical hardware configuration in the form of a computer workstation.

The parts of the computer program which are required by the CPU for it to operate are loaded into the system RAM, the remainder being transferred to user-RAM. As RAM is erased on switch-off, it is important to remember to save the output produced for each session of computer use. It

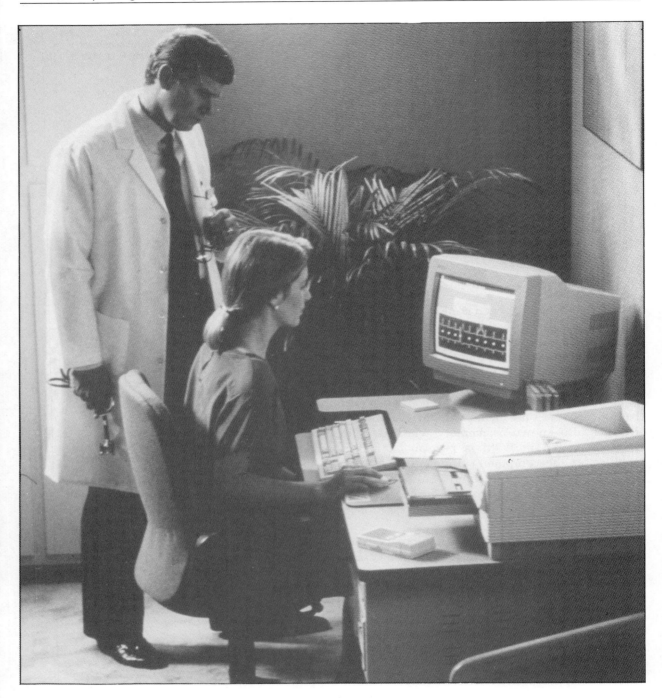

Figure 2.2(b) Computer
hardware: PC-based halter
system in use. (By courtesy of
Hewlett-Packard Ltd.)

is good practice in any case to save (back-up) data at regular intervals, since even a short disruption or spike (glitch) in the electricity supply may be sufficient to erase RAM, or input may be corrupted by a wrong key stroke.

2.6.2 Software

Applications software consists of wordprocessing packages, databases and spreadsheets as well as programming languages such as BASIC, PASCAL and C. The operating system is needed to prevent the user from having to program at the lowest level by means of binary computer instructions. Examples of operating systems include the 'Disk Operating System' (DOS) used with IBM and compatible computers, and 'UNIX' used with more powerful multiple-task computers.

It can be argued that we use the decimal system of arithmetic because we have ten fingers. Similarly, a computer uses the binary system (which has two digits 0 and 1) because these states can be represented by the presence or absence of an electronic pulse. The 0s and 1s are termed BInary digiTs (or BITS) and eight BITS comprise one BYTE. Each byte has sufficient states to represent a character on the keyboard. This can be seen as follows:

1 BIT can represent two characters $(2)^1$
(0, 1)
2 BITS can represent four characters $(2)^2$
(00, 01, 10, 11)
3 BITS can represent eight characters $(2)^3$
(000, 001, 010, 011, 100, 101, 110, 111)

Similarly 8 BITS can represent 2^8 (256) characters, but in practice the zero character is omitted. Many character states are left unassigned on a computer keyboard.

Bytes are also used to determine the storage capacity of computer equipment measured in terms of the number of bytes of RAM, since this determines the space available for holding the applications software. The original IBM personal computer had 64,000 bytes of RAM (64 kB). Programs have become more complex and RAM-size dependent, forcing computer manufacturers to investigate ways of increasing the size of RAM while keeping computer prices competitive. It is now not uncommon to have available 4 000 000 bytes (4 MB) or more of RAM, with powerful personal computers holding up to 64 MB of RAM.

Electrical circuits are available which can 'add' or 'subtract' the pulses which mimic the operation of the binary system of arithmetic. Hardwired computer instructions are simply various configurations of these circuits. Although more inflexible in their operation, hardwired special purpose computers are employed to obtain the fast speed of operation for defined procedures, as in some areas of medical image-signal processing.

2.6.3 Storage

No matter how many megabytes of RAM are resident in a computer, as soon as the power supply is switched off, the programs are lost unless temporary back-up is provided. This can be catastrophic if switch-off was not anticipated. One way to prevent loss of data is to arrange a timely storage of results from a computer program. Looking back for several years a set of punch cards or punched paper tape was used where the convention employed was that the presence of a hole represented a '1' and the absence of a hole represented a '0'. Optical readers could scan the cards or tape and decode the pattern of holes or spaces. This process was relatively slow and has now been superseded by the availability of magnetic media, originally magnetic cassette tape and then by magnetic disks.

The shape of the magnetic media changed because rotating disk drives could locate a particular place on a disk far more rapidly than is possible with a serial medium such as magnetic tape. Manufacturers have agreed on two standard sizes of computer disks: the 'floppy' $5\frac{1}{4}$ inch and the more robust $3\frac{1}{2}$ inch disk. Typically, 1.4 megabytes of data can be stored on each $3\frac{1}{2}$ inch disk and 1.2 megabytes on each floppy disk. This information allows calculation of how many patients' records can be stored on one disk and this is particularly important when recording on-line data. Adequate data-storage provision is vital.

Although floppy disks are currently the most common storage device, optical disk storage is rapidly becoming available, for example in the storage of ultrasound and X-ray medical images. The technology used is similar to that of audio compact disks (CDs) and is known as CD-ROM. An advantage of this technique is that the storage capacity can be increased to giga-bytes allowing the storage of much more data per disk. One of the drawbacks of CD-ROM, which will shortly be overcome by the general introduction of read/write optical disks, is that data once saved cannot then be retrieved (hence the significance of read-only memory). Paradoxically, for the purposes of medical records, this may be a valuable attribute since for medico-legal and security reasons it should not be possible to tamper with the data.

2.6.4 Communications

Communications protocols are required when data is to be sent from computer to computer or from computer to printer. Data can be transmitted in one of two ways, either in parallel or serial form. When in parallel mode, all eight BITS which make up each BYTE (and therefore a keyboard character) are sent simultaneously. This requires the use of 8 cables and is the better option in terms of speed of transmission when the data link is relatively short, e.g. within an intensive care unit. In serial mode, the eight BITS are sent sequentially. This has to be slower than the parallel mode although there is the advantage that only one cable is needed. This cable can be an optical fibre cable, coaxial cable or a twisted pair of conductors depending on circumstances such as the speed of the link, but it may under special circumstances be possible to use some form of telephone line. This makes it feasible to send and receive data over distances of many miles and with satellite transmission over thousands of miles.

The digital data output from the computer is not directly compatible with telephone-line transmission and has to be modified (modulated) in a special fashion to suit the characteristics of the telephone network. Once the data are received at the other end of the link, the incoming signals must be demodulated before being presented to the receiving computer. This MODulation-DEModulation process is performed by devices known as modems. Telephone modems are in regular use with computer-data networks. For example, ECGs can be acquired from patients in Boston Massachusetts and transmitted to a computer for automatic interpretation in Atlanta Georgia – a distance of nearly 2000 miles (Tomkins, W. J. and Webster, J. G. (1981) *Design of Microcomputer-based Medical Instrumentation*, Englewood Cliffs, Prentice Hall).

Another form of computer communication occurs with what are termed 'networked systems'. A computer network comprises a number of computers, each having its own data-processing capability and linked together to share one large central disk-storage facility, known as a file server. The networks can be wide area networks (WANs) or local area networks (LANs) depending on the distances involved between each computer. WANs are used between satellite hospitals and clinics and a major hospital or between satellite laboratories and a central pathology laboratory.

Of more interest in high dependency situations are LANs. An intensive care unit may have several computer-based patient monitors linked to a central nursing station by a LAN. In most cases the file server of the LAN is linked to the hospital information system (HIS), which is a larger LAN, from which it is possible to obtain patient-demographic data as well as data from other departments such as out-patient clinics and laboratories.

One form of local area network is based on 'carrier sense multiple access with collision detection' (CSMA/CD). Fortunately, this technique is usually known by the name 'Ethernet' after its first operational example. The Ethernet network was developed by the Xerox Corporation in the USA in the early 1970s. Success for this method of computer inter-communication was guaranteed when Ethernet became an international standard in 1984.

The configuration for an Ethernet network is similar to the bus network shown in Figure 2.3c. It utilizes a coaxial cable bus terminated at both ends for communication at data rates of approximately 10 megabits per second. The quoted data rate indicates the amount of data which can be transmitted per second, where 10 megabits is roughly equivalent to 1.4 million bytes per second. This means that 1.4 million alphanumeric characters can be transmitted in each second. This is sufficiently fast to capture all the clinical data required for many tens of patients as it has been estimated that the data rate per patient in an intensive care unit is approximately 2000 bytes per second. When a message is transmitted from any computer on an Ethernet network it is passed on to all the other computers connected to the network. As the maximum separation of the computers can be 2.5 kilometres and the maximum number of computers connected to an Ethernet bus is 1024 there is a need to copy, or amplify, the transmitted signal. There are also special protocols which sense 'collisions'

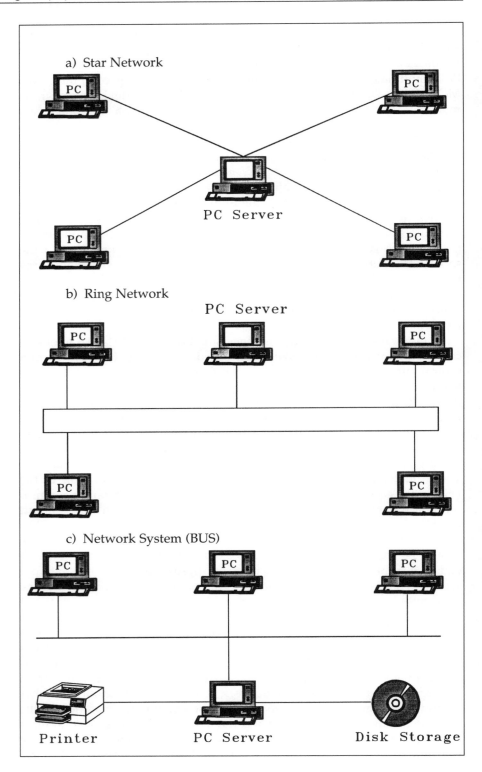

Figure 2.3 Comparison between a) Star, b) Ring and c) Bus configuration network systems.

in data and prevent clinical data from being corrupted. Each device connected to the Ethernet has a unique physical address on the network which allows the collection of audit information such as bed occupancy.

There are several different types (topologies) of network. The most popular are the star, the ring and the bus (Busbar) configurations, which are compared in Figure 2.3. Even in LANs, the computers may be geographically relatively remote. Hence, special cabling is required to prevent corruption or loss of data. A popular choice is a network based on Ethernet cables. These are electrically shielded cables in order to minimize outside interference from other electrical sources such as lifts and hospital communications systems. In the star network, the central file server is attached to a multiplexer which acts as a form of multi-way switch and controls the flow of data between each of the participating computers in sequence.

This arrangement is well-suited to expansion, the limit being set by the speed of the multiplexer. The ring network is based on the use of a continual run of cable where each computer 'passes on' the signals and commands. Here there is a need for a signal amplifier in the line to prevent the attenuation of data or commands. The bus network uses a central cable (Busbar in electrical power engineering terminology) to which each computer is connected. The central file server is also attached to the bus, so that any one computer can communicate with the file server or indeed with any other computer which is connected to the bus. It is this latter type of network which holds out much promise for data networks in clinical situations.

The Institute of Electrical and Electronic Engineers (IEEE) in the United States is in the process of producing a standard definition to cover the requirements of a 'medical information bus'. This is an attractive concept, since if every manufacturer of medical instrumentation adopted this proposed standard, it would become possible to connect any computer or microprocessor-based equipment (ventilator, blood-gas analyser, patient monitor) to the medical information bus, allowing maximum integration of patient data from which to optimize patient management and care.

3 Physiological pressure measurements

3.1 Introduction

The need to measure pressures such as arterial and venous blood pressures using an invasive technique and airway pressure when an automatic lung ventilator is in operation is commonplace in patient monitoring during major surgery and intensive care. In urodynamic studies pressures such as bladder and rectal pressures may be required to be measured and recorded on a chart recorder. Hence, pressure transducers which convert physiological pressures into a corresponding analogue electrical signal form an important component of medical instrumentation used by operating room and intensive care unit staff. While disposable pressure transducers are available, the majority of pressure transducers are reuseable. This implies that they must be readily capable of being sterilized without being damaged. They are accurate devices which need to be used with respect, i.e. not dropped and not overloaded to outside the pressure limits specified by the manufacturer.

Most pressure transducers are designed to be operated outside the patient's body. On the one hand, this may pose problems with the physical connection of the transducer to the site of the pressure to be measured. On the other, the transducer is immediately available for purposes such as establishing a reference (baseline) pressure or for calibration. The tubing connecting the transducer to the site of the pressure to be measured is filled with heparinized sterile physiological saline for blood-pressure measurements but is air filled for airway-pressure measurements.

There are also pressure transducers which have been specifically designed for use within the body, e.g. within the heart or major blood vessels. These are supplied mounted at the end of a suitable gauge cardiac catheter. The constructional requirements are demanding. The transducer must not damage the interior of the vessels through which it passes, and it must have a stable calibration inside the body, since a recalibration involves the removal of the transducer from the patient. There is also a need for the non-invasive measurement of arterial blood pressure in patients whose condition does not warrant the insertion of an arterial line and the use of a pressure transducer. Numerous other situations dealing with obstetric patients and volunteers also require non-invasive blood-pressure measurements which can be carried out if need be over periods of several hours.

3.2 Strain-gauge pressure transducers

Many suppliers of patient-monitoring equipment use silicon diaphragm strain gauge-pressure transducers designed for use outside the patient's body. Pressure is defined as force per unit area. The application of the pressure to be measured to one side of a diaphragm causes the diaphragm to move slightly in the opposite direction and in a well-designed transducer the amplitude of the resulting small motion is linearly related to the applied pressure. The motion of the diaphragm can be measured by making use of strain-gauge technology.

Referring to Figure 3.1 the diaphragm is mounted at one end of the transducer's housing which contains the circuit components of a strain-gauge bridge. The interior of the housing bounded by the rear of the diaphragm is usually at atmospheric pressure and this constitutes the reference pressure against which are measured changes occurring in the physiological pressure of interest. In some applications, such as the measurement of intrinsic bladder pressure, it is necessary to measure the difference between two pressures such as bladder and rectal pressure. For this purpose a differential pressure transducer is used where one pressure is applied to the front of the diaphragm and one to the back.

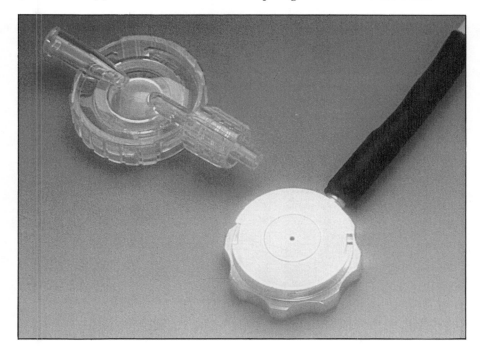

Figure 3.1 Strain gauge physiological pressure transducer with a pressure range of −20 to +300 mmHg, a maximum overpressure of 10 000 mmHg, a sensitivity of 50 microvolts per volt per 10 mmHg, maximum excitation of 15 V a.c. or d.c. and a typical resonant frequency of 300 Hz. (Courtesy of SensoNor a.s.)

The diaphragm is made from silicon which is physically strong and chemically inert. Silicon is also attractive because it can be used as the substrate for fabricating semiconductor strain gauges which are bonded on to the diaphragm's rear surface. The front surface of the diaphragm forms one face of a small volume chamber known as the cuvette or dome which is fitted with two connections and via them a pair of stopcocks. These permit the pressure to be measured, or reference/calibration pressures to be applied to the cuvette or for the cuvette to be flushed out.

Traditionally the transducer housing was cylindrical in shape and was mounted in a clamp attached to a board supporting the patient's arm or to a drip stand. However, in the latter case a restless patient can move his arm and loosen the tubing connecting his circulation to the transducer and this could lead to haemorrhage. Flat transducers can be taped to the patient's skin so that no relative movement can occur between the patient and the transducer.

3.2.1 The strain-gauge bridge

When a length of wire is stretched, not only does its length increase but it becomes thinner and its cross-sectional area decreases. Both of these actions cause an increase in the electrical resistance of the wire. Conversely, if a wire is shortened its resistance will decrease. Referring to Figure 3.2, it is possible to select areas on the rear of a transducer's diaphragm where strain gauges will be either stretched or shortened. The four gauges can be used as two pairs (one stretching, one shortening) to form the four arms of a Wheatstone bridge circuit, Figure 3.3. Because all

Figure 3.2 The action of strain gauges located on the rear surface of the silicon diaphragm of a pressure transducer to form a strain gauge full bridge.

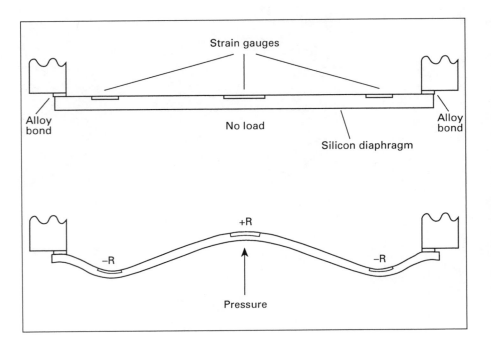

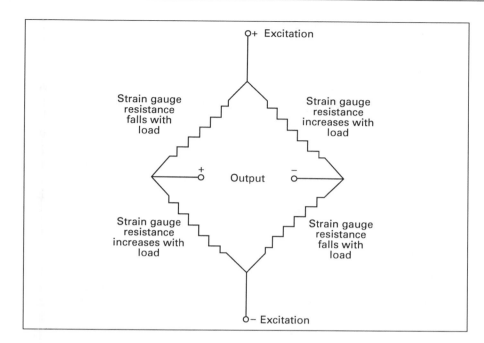

+ Excitation

Strain gauge
resistance
falls with
load

Strain gauge
resistance
increases with
load

+   −
Output

Strain gauge
resistance
increases with
load

Strain gauge
resistance
falls with
load

− Excitation

Figure 3.3 Circuit of a strain
gauge full bridge.

four arms change their resistance when pressure is applied across the diaphragm, this arrangement is called a strain-gauge full bridge. The bridge can be energized from a stable d.c. supply or a stable audio-frequency source. In the case of a.c. excitation this typically would be 5 volts r.m.s. at 3906 Hz. This frequency can be selected by a tuned filter which will reject frequencies which are multiples of 50 Hz or 60 Hz, thus helping to eliminate mains frequency interference.

In practice the gauges are not made from wire but from silicon semiconductor material because of the increase in sensitivity which results, perhaps by a factor of 50.This is largely due to the resulting distortion of the crystalline structure of the silicon. However, the semiconductor gauges are more temperature sensitive and show a greater non-linearity than would wire gauges. Several silicon gauges are laid down on the rear of the silicon diaphragm by means of integrated circuit fabrication technology and the best set of four selected on test. The diaphragm is clamped only at its periphery by alloying to a metal ring having the same coefficient of expansion. Additional external and variable resistances are built into the complete bridge circuit so that the operator can balance the bridge to give a zero output voltage when the pressures on either side of the diaphragm are equal.

If the pressure on one side of the diaphragm increases relative to that on the other the output signal goes positive, while if the pressure decreases relative to the other side for d.c. excitation the output signal goes negative. Hence, the magnitude of the pressure difference across the diaphragm is proportional to the magnitude of the output signal and an increase or decrease of the applied pressure is shown by the polarity of the output signal. The absolute amplitude of the output signal when the bridge unbalances is proportional to the magnitude of the excitation voltage.

Manufacturers of patient monitors quote the sensitivity of transducers suitable for use with their monitors and which are likely to have been supplied from another manufacturer. A typical transducer sensitivity would be 50 microvolts per volt excitation per 10 mm mercury pressure plus or minus 1%. The output signal is approximately linearly related to the excitation when the deformation of the diaphragm under the influence of the pressure to be measured is small. This is evident from the fact that the output signal is only one twenty thousandth of the excitation for a typical silicon diaphragm transducer. During construction a batch of gauges will be adjusted at the factory to all have this sensitivity so that they can easily be interchanged.

3.2.2 Transducer cuvettes

The transducer's cuvette is fabricated from a rigid transparent plastic material and is attached to the front of the transducer housing by means of a knurled screw ring or partial turn-locking device to enable the cuvette to be conveniently removed from the housing and diaphragm for cleaning or replacement, Figure 3.4. The cuvette is provided with a pair of female luer-lock connectors to which may be attached stopcocks and plastic

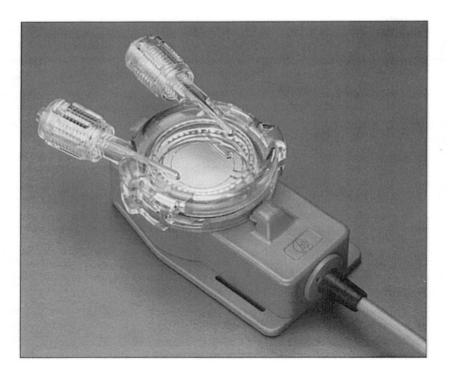

Figure 3.4 Hewlett Packard Model 1290C Quartz Pressure Transducer. (Courtesy Hewlett Packard Company.)

catheters/cannulas as required. The cuvette moulding is often dome-shaped and is commonly called the 'dome'. It should be designed to have a small volume which is readily visible from its exterior so that the presence of a small bubble, when the cuvette is filled with sterile saline, can be easily detected.

The polished front surface of the diaphragm must be handled with care and not subjected to cleaning with abrasive compounds. The cuvette attached to the transducer can be chemically sterilized using a sterilizing solution recommended by the manufacturer. After the sterilizing solution has been left in place for the necessary length of time, the cuvette and stopcocks should be well flushed through with sterile physiological saline solution and the stopcocks shut.

Disposable cuvettes are available which are single use 'one-trip' devices. The bottom of the disposable cuvette consists of a slack plastic diaphragm which sits on top of the transducer's diaphragm. There is now less risk of cross-infection between patients because a new sterile dome is used for each patient and the slack plastic diaphragm also provides additional electrical insulation with respect to leakage currents from the transducer reaching the patient. Packs of ten disposable domes sterilized by gamma radiation can be supplied.

3.2.3 Transducer 'plumbing'

The connection from one of the transducer's stopcocks to the patient is normally via a cannula or a catheter. It is important when measuring blood pressures that all the tubing plus the cuvette is filled completely with sterile heparinized physiological saline solution. Because air is very compressible relative to saline, the presence of even a small air bubble will significantly dampen an arterial pressure tracing, since the arterial pulsating pressure acts on the bubble rather than on the transducer's diaphragm. Bubbles can be removed by flushing the system through with sterile saline from a syringe via the second stopcock. It is vitally important that the distal stopcock is not closed during this process. A small diameter syringe can generate high pressures sufficient to permanently damage the transducer. A syringe of less than 10 ml capacity should not be used for this reason.

Damping of the blood-pressure waveform can also occur if a blood clot partially occludes the distal tip of the catheter or cannula. An inexperienced observer may think that the cardiac action of the patient has deteriorated rather than that the tracing is an artifact consequent upon the presence of a clot. When blood-pressure monitoring over several hours is required, it is usual to continuously perfuse the arterial line with heparinized saline at a rate of typically 4 ml per hour from an elevated drip bag or bottle or from a plastic bag which has been pressurized by wrapping it around with an inflated cuff. A restrictor may be used to set the flow of saline and disposable assemblies are available containing the restrictor and connectors. The low flow rate of saline does not affect the fidelity of the pressure tracing.

3.2.4 Frequency response of the transducer-catheter system

The column of fluid connecting the transducer to the site of the blood pressure limits the range of frequencies which can be faithfully reproduced by the complete system. Factors involved include the inertia of the mass of fluid in the tubing, the resistance of the fluid in the tube, the diameter and length of the tubing and the stiffness of the transducer's diaphragm. For the highest frequency response, a short, wide bore tube should be used with a transducer having a stiff diaphragm. However, clinical conditions usually determine the length and gauge of the catheter or cannula which may be used. The greater the stiffness of the transducer's diaphragm, the less is its sensitivity. In terms of diaphragm stiffness, transducer manufacturers quote the volume displacement of the device in cubic millimetres displacement per 100 mm Hg pressure applied. For a pressure transducer with a volume displacement of 0.2 cubic millimetres per 100 mm Hg connected to a one metre long catheter of internal diameter 1.5 mm and filled with physiological saline, the frequency response is 47 Hz which would well cover heart rates of 120 beats per minute.

The damping of the catheter-transducer system is important because if the system is underdamped an overshoot may appear on steeply rising portions of the pressure waveform, whereas if it is overdamped sharply rising peaks may be underestimated. For high fidelity recordings the components of the complete pressure-recording system may have to be selected in accordance with the manufacturer's recommendations to give the optimum damping.

3.3 Capacitive blood-pressure transducers

An interesting development by Hewlett Packard is the fused quartz capacitive physiological pressure transducer, Figure 3.4. It consists of a quartz body 6.4 mm thick and a diaphragm 1.25 mm thick. The diaphragm and body are brazed together using a tin-gold alloy. Quartz is used to attain a small temperature coefficient of sensitivity. The body of the transducer has etched into it a shallow cavity which is only 10 micrometres deep and has one electrode at the bottom of the cavity. A second electrode is located on the rear of the diaphragm. The two electrodes, together with the gap which separates them, form a parallel plate electrode capacitor. As pressure is applied to the front surface of the diaphragm, this moves backwards and the spacing between the electrodes decreases causing the capacitance of the capacitor to increase.

The body of the transducer contains a miniature 8.4 kHz audio-frequency circuit which produces an output voltage which is linearly proportional to the applied pressure. It uses a bridge circuit to measure the change in capacitance between the variable capacitor of the transducer and that of a reference capacitor contained within the transducer. The construction resembles that of a wristwatch so that it can easily be taped to the skin of a patient.

The transducer can be energized with 5 to 10 V d.c. or with 3.5 to 8 V r.m.s. a.c. from 1 kHz to 5 kHz. The leakage current is less than 5 microamperes at 120 V r.m.s. 60 Hz and the device will withstand up to 16 000 volts peak defibrillator pulses applied from the fluid column to all the connector pins shorted together. The possible pressure range is –50 to +300mm Hg, the volume displacement is 0.2 cubic millimetres per 100 mm Hg and the device can withstand –400 mm Hg to +4000 mm Hg. The output sensitivity is standardized to 50 microvolts per volt excitation per 10 mm Hg pressure. The quartz transducer can be sterilized by ethylene oxide gas or disinfected with liquid agents such as gluteraldehyde. Disposable domes are also used.

3.4 Catheter-tip pressure transducers

Miniature strain-gauge transducers have been developed which can be mounted at the tip of a 6 French gauge cardiac catheter 1 metre long. Such devices are both relatively delicate and expensive and must be handled with care. The choice of materials used in their construction is important since the baseline and the pressure calibration must not change significantly while the transducer is recording in the patient's heart or vasculature. If this happens, the transducer would have to be withdrawn for a recalibration.

Because there is no long fluid column involved, the frequency response of the catheter-tip transducer can extend to beyond 4 kHz. Thus, in addition to pressure recording with the amplifier bandwidth limited to 0 to 100 Hz, a second channel having a much wider audio-frequency bandwidth can be used with the transducer also acting as a microphone, to record heart sounds. Filters separate the blood-pressure signals from the phonocardiogram signals.

More sophisticated forms of catheter-tip transducers are available. There may be two pressure recording elements spaced apart so that the pressure gradient existing across a heart valve can be monitored. There may also be a flow transducer to monitor blood-flow patterns and a thermistor to monitor blood temperature. This type of multi-transducer catheter is guided into place via X-ray fluoroscopy in a cardiac catheterization laboratory.

3.5 Calibration of pressure transducers

The calibration of a pressure transducer designed for use outside of the patient is accomplished by first closing the stopcock leading to the catheter/cannula and opening the second stopcock first to atmospheric (room) pressure to allow the baseline of the recording to be set. The second stopcock is then turned to put the transducer's cuvette in communication with a source of known pressures. This is usually a mercury manometer or a column of sterile saline to measure the calibration pressures which can be generated by means of a manual sphygmomanometer.

Another possibility is to use a commercial pressure calibrator in which a manually operated piston and cylinder generate pressures which are read by an accurately calibrated digital-pressure transducer whose pressure reading is shown on a digital liquid-crystal display. Catheter-tip pressure transducers are calibrated by passing the catheter through a watertight seal into a vessel containing water at body temperature and to whose interior can be applied known pressures from a sphygmomanometer.

3.6 The choice of a reference pressure level

Blood pressures are quoted in respect of a reference plane which is usually taken to be at the level of the patient's heart. If the transducer is mounted on a stand which permits it to be raised or lowered, it can easily be adjusted so that the transducer's diaphragm is at mid-heart level. The question of the plane from which measurements are taken becomes more important when measuring lower value pressures such as the central venous pressure, and note of changes in the patient's position may need to be taken into account.

3.7 Non-invasive blood-pressure measurements

Non-invasive blood-pressure (NIBP) monitoring is widely offered as part of comprehensive patient-monitoring systems. It is attractive for patients whose severity of condition does not warrant invasive measurements. Essentially a compressor is arranged, on command, to inflate a pressurized cuff wrapped around an upper arm to inflate the bladder of the cuff to a pressure which is above that of the patient's systolic blood pressure. A pressure-leak valve is then activated and this is designed to provide a linear fall in the cuff pressure. Korotkoff sounds occur when the systolic pressure is reached and these persist as the pressure in the cuff falls, until at the diastolic pressure they become muffled and then disappear. The presence of Korotkoff sounds can be detected by means of a crystal microphone placed beneath the cuff, but problems can be experienced due to artifacts produced by movement of the patient's arm.

Patient-monitoring systems utilize the oscillometry method with a double cuff. The principle of operation is the sensing of the sudden increase in the volume oscillations of the cuff which occurs at the systolic pressure and the sudden decrease in their amplitude which occurs at the diastolic pressure. Consider the upper cuff nearer the patient's shoulder than the lower cuff. With both cuffs inflated to above the systolic pressure, pulsations from the artery will reach the upper but not the lower cuff. As the pressure is reduced to below systolic, pulsations reach the lower cuff but after a delay. The delay is due to the inertia of the column of blood and the arterial wall. When diastolic pressure is reached, the artery is fully open and there is no delay in the pulsations detected with each cuff. By monitoring the presence or absence of pulsations and the time delay both

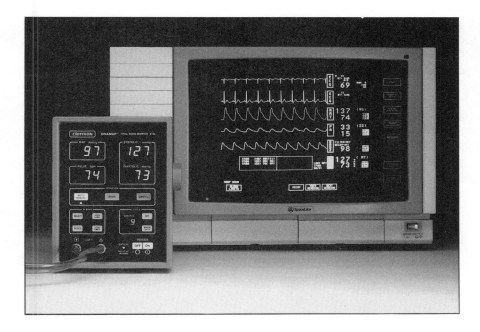

Figure 3.5 Portable non-invasive blood-pressure system. The unit can operate for up to 6 hours from its rechargeable battery measuring blood pressures every five minutes. It is shown with a patient monitor. (Courtesy Critikon and Spacelabs.)

the systolic and diastolic pressures can be read from a calibrated pressure transducer contained in the monitor, Figure 3.5.

Sapinski, A. (1992) 'Standard algorithm of blood-pressure measurement by the oscillometric method' *Medical and Biological Engineering and Computing*, **30**, 671, discusses the derivation of the systolic, mean and diastolic pressures by the oscillometric technique. Referring to Figure 3.6, as the cuff pressure is gradually decreased from above the systolic pressure, a characteristic change in the pulse waveform is observed at pressures in the cuff corresponding with the systolic (SP) and mean pressure (MP). In one commercial system (the Dinamap) the systolic pressure is taken as that pressure at which a sudden increase in the pressure oscillations occurs. The mean pressure is taken as that at which the maximum oscillation occurs and the diastolic pressure (DP) is taken as that at which the first sudden drop in the oscillation occurs. For a greater accuracy, Sapinski (1992) takes the peak amplitude at the mean pressure to be 100%, the systolic pressure as the point corresponding with the preceding 40% of the maximum and the diastolic pressure as the

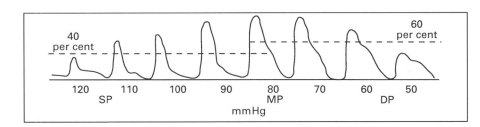

Figure 3.6 The relationships between the oscillometric cuff pressure and the systolic, mean and diastolic pressures. (From Sapinski 1992 with permission.)

point corresponding with the following 60% of the maximum amplitude of oscillation. These ratios result from the formula Mean Pressure = Diastolic Pressure + 0.4 Pulse Pressure, where the Pulse Pressure = (Systolic–Diastolic).

Typical blood-pressure ranges measured would be for adults up to 260 mmHg systolic and up to 240 mmHg diastolic. The interval between successive measurements can be set from 1 to 60 minutes with a measurement time of less than 45 seconds. A variety of cuffs is available for adult and child use and also a thigh cuff. The controlling microprocessor provides watchdog timer facilities for the software and a hardware timer to monitor the cuff pressure and automatically open pressure bleed valves after 3 minutes of inflation. Automatic cuff deflation occurs if the cuff pressure exceeds 315 mmHg. Modern non-invasive blood-pressure monitors make use of miniature quiet compressors so that an NIBP module can easily be mounted in a rack along with other modules.

The monitoring of body temperature

4

4.1 Introduction

The measurement of body temperature is very commonly performed since an elevated body temperature may be associated with an infection and a depressed value may be indicative of shock. In the past, body temperatures have been quoted on both the Fahrenheit and Centigrade temperature scales. However, present practice is to use the degree Celsius, as this is the SI unit of temperature and is numerically the same as the degree Centigrade.

It is traditionally measured by means of a mercury-in-glass thermometer. In the United Kingdom clinical thermometers are each checked for accuracy at the Test House of the British Standards Institution. Although compact and accurate, clinical thermometers can only be read close to the site of measurement and the constituent materials of glass and mercury can represent a health hazard if the thermometer is broken. It has been argued that rectal temperatures should not be taken because of the risk of thermometer breakage. However, Morley, C. J., Hewson, P. H., Thornton, A. J. and Cole, T. J. (1992) 'Axillary and rectal temperature measurements in infants and young children' *Archives of Diseases of Childhood*, **67**, 122–5 estimate the risk of rectal perforation by a thermometer as less than one in two million. The problems of broken thermometers are discussed in a Safety Action Bulletin (March 1992) issued by the Medical Devices Directorate of the UK's Department of Health. Instructions to staff who have to deal with broken thermometers must include information for the complete removal of mercury.

Spirit-based thermometers can also produce a hazard if broken. The Bulletin provides an interesting description of the problems associated with a broken Six's pattern Maximum-Minimum thermometer used for checking vaccine-storage conditions in a hospital ward. The thermometer contained a spirit mixture comprising equal parts of wood creosote and toluene. The spread of the pungent odour necessitated the evacuation of more than 30 patients from the ward. Alternative methods include liquid crystal temperature indicators for skin-temperature monitoring and thermistor-temperature probes used as sensors as part of a patient-monitor system. Thermocouples offer the advantage of a miniature measuring element which can be contained within a hypodermic needle but are usually only encountered in experimental studies.

Clarke, S. (1992) 'Use of thermometers in general practice', *British Medical Journal*, **304**, 961–3, draws attention to the need to allow a period of 3 minutes for a mercury-in-glass clinical thermometer's reading to stabilize. This is in contrast with electronic thermometers which take less than one minute to provide a final reading (thermistor probes without a substantial metal sheath). Keeley, D. (1992) 'Taking infant's temperatures', *British Medical Journal*, **304**, 932–3 states that a mercury-in-glass thermometer in place for one minute will very occasionally miss an appreciable fever while an electronic thermometer can be read in seconds. Keeley (1992) cites several studies which have shown the unreliability of axillary temperatures in children. Axillary and rectal temperatures were shown to differ inconsistently by up to 3 degrees Celsius.

It must also be remembered that the presence of food and drink can affect all oral measurements of temperature. There is also an effect of circadian rhythm on body temperature and cyclic effects of gonadal steroids on the core temperature of pre-menopausal women. A paper by Czeisler, C. A., Dumont, Marie, Duffy, Jeanne F., Steinberg, J. D., Richardson, G. S., Brown, E. N., Sanchez, R., Rios, C. D. and Ronda, J. M. (1992) 'Association of sleep-wake habits in older people with changes in output of circadian pacemaker', The *Lancet*, **340**, 933–6 quotes a mean body temperature of 37.0 degrees Celsius for a group of 27 young men (18–31 years) and a mean endogenous circadian temperature oscillation of 0.28 degrees in comparison with 36.89 and 0.17 degrees Celsius for a group of 11 old men (65–85 years).

Tissue-temperature measurements are important in the technique of hyperthermia (thermotherapy) for the treatment of tumours in which the aim of the therapy is to produce tissue temperatures between 42.5 and 43 degrees Celsius for 30 to 60 minutes per treatment and 10 to 15 treatments may be required. The methods employed to produce tissue heating are: the application of ultrasound energy in the frequency range 0.3 to 3 MHz; radiofrequency power at frequencies below 300 MHz and microwave energy at frequencies of 300 to 2450 MHz. It is claimed that transrectal heating of the prostate gland by microwaves at 1000 MHz is effective in reducing the symptoms of prostatic outflow obstruction and increasing urine flow rates in men. The treatment aims to heat the prostate to about 43 degrees Celsius via a rectal probe together with water cooling of the rectal wall in order to avoid necrosis. An alternative technique delivers microwave energy to the prostate via a urethral probe. This avoids damage to the rectal wall and also appears to be more capable of generating a symmetrical heating of the prostate. It is claimed that one or two treatments on an out-patient basis, each of one to three hours duration, will produce an immediate benefit to the patient. See Carter, S., Patel, A., Reddy, P., Royer, P. and Ramsay, J. (1991) 'Single-session transurethral microwave thermotherapy for the treatment of benign prostatic obstruction', *Journal of Endocrinology*, **5**, 137–44; Ogden, C. W., Reddy, P., Johnson,

H., Ramsay, J. W. A. and Carter, S. St. C. (1993) 'Sham versus transurethral microwave thermotherapy in patients with symptoms of benign prostatic bladder outflow obstruction', *The Lancet*, **341**, 14–17.

Whole-body heating combined with chemotherapy is also employed using radiant electrical heating or immersion in a bath of hot water. A difficult problem which arises in undertaking hyperthermia for superficial or deeper lesions occurs with the absence of a uniform temperature distribution with the tissues being heated and the need to accurately monitor temperatures inside large and geometrically complex tumours. Thermistor probes inserted into the tissue are used and only a limited number of these can be located within the mass. The report by Green, I. (1991) 'Hyperthermia alone or combined with chemotherapy for the treatment of cancer', Health Technology Assessment Reports No. 2, Department of Health and Human Services, Rockville, Maryland MD 20887, USA, states that the usefulness of this modality of cancer therapy remains unclear.

4.2 The concept of core and peripheral temperatures

The simple term body temperature is not sufficiently precise for a number of patient-monitoring applications where a knowledge of the core (deep body) temperature and peripheral (skin) temperature may be required. An example occurs in the case of cardiac surgery under profound hypothermia where a knowledge of the temperature of the heart is of importance as an aid in avoiding the production of cardiac arrhythmias during rewarming. This may be approximated by the temperature in the oesophagus at heart level which may differ from the rectal temperature by 2 or 3 degrees Celsius.

As an indication of deep body temperature, suitably designed temperature probes can be positioned in the mouth or rectum. The onset of peripheral circulation shutdown can be detected by an increasing difference between the deep body and peripheral temperatures. It is for this reason that patient monitors often provide the facility to monitor two temperatures and sometimes the difference between them. It has also been shown that changes in the temperature measured of the big toe follows changes occurring in the patient's cardiac output. Randall, N. J., Bond, K., Macaulay, J. and Steer, P. J. (1991) 'Measuring fetal and maternal temperature differentials: a probe for clinical use during labour', *Journal of Biomedical Engineering*, **13**, 481–5 describe the measurement of temperature differentials existing between mother and foetus during labour.

Greenleaf, J. E. and Castle, B. L. (1972) 'External auditory canal temperature as an estimate of core temperature', *Journal of Applied Physiology*, **32**, 194–8, showed that the external auditory canal temperature does not estimate core temperature but may be used to estimate mean body temperature. At least one medical emergency-helicopter service has found the external auditory canal temperature of value in the assessment of casualties attended away from hospital.

4.3 Temperature Sensors

Patient monitoring requires the availability of a variety of temperature probes. Some will need to be waterproof and fitted with a stainless steel outer cover to facilitate cleaning after insertion into the rectum. The outer surface must be smooth to prevent injury to the patient. The thermal inertia of the covering will give rise to a relatively long response time of several seconds which is unlikely to present problems in practice. However, a fast response time is required in a sensor to follow changes in respired air temperature. A flat sensor is needed for skin temperature measurements. A typical temperature monitoring channel for a patient-monitoring system based upon a thermistor probe supplied by the American Yellow Springs Instrument Company covers the temperature range 0 to 50 degrees Celsius with a resolution of 0.1 degrees and an accuracy of plus or minus 0.3 degrees. The maximum current leakage from the probe is less than 10 microamperes.

4.4 Liquid crystal thermometers

These consist of strips of crystalline material chosen so that they each change colour at a predetermined temperature. A scale with increments of 2 degrees Celsius is placed adjacent to the strips. The thermometer is placed on the patient's forehead and the strip which corresponds with the patient's skin temperature at the time appears to show a distinctive colour, perhaps orange, with the strips on either side showing a different colour. The device provides a convenient method for the routine visible monitoring of temperature trends in patients whose precise core temperature does not need to be monitored. However, Clark (1992) cites reports which state that liquid crystal 'fever strips' are inaccurate. Liquid crystal temperature indicators are usually backed by a sheet of plastic which must be removed before the device is affixed to the patient's skin, or a low reading will result.

4.5 Thermistors

A thermistor is a THERMally sensitive resISTOR, that is a resistor whose resistance alters markedly with changes of its ambient temperature. A thermistor is also known as a negative temperature coefficient (NTC) resistor since its resistance falls markedly with an increase in its temperature. In practice, a thermistor designed for use in a body-temperature probe might consist of a small bead of semiconductor material sealed into the tip of a thin glass envelope for protection. Platinum leads are fused into the bead and led out of the envelope via metal-to-glass seals. The bead material could consist of a mixture of nickel, cobalt and manganese oxides fused together in a furnace during production. A typical bead resistance might be 2000 ohms at 20 degrees Celsius which would fall to 1400 ohms at 40 degrees Celsius. Each bead is subject to a carefully controlled ageing process during manufacture to ensure a stability of calibration.

Rugged thermistors for use in areas such as the monitoring of the temperature of a water bath can use a thermistor made of semiconductor polycrystalline metal oxide ceramic. Between 0 and 70 degrees Celsius the measuring accuracy is 0.2 degrees and the response can be less than two seconds. The variation of the thermistor resistance with temperature is inherently non-linear. In order to ensure that thermistor probes of the same type have the same sensitivity and linearity characteristics so that they can be interchanged, the manufacturer places additional conventional resistances in parallel and in series with the probe inside the probe housing during test to linearize the calibration and standardize the sensitivity. The high sensitivity of thermistors enables them to be used as one arm of a Wheatstone bridge circuit fed from a stabilized voltage supply.

4.6 Thermocouples

A thermocouple comprises an electrical circuit made from wires of two different materials. Typically one would be copper and the other constantan (an alloy containing 60% copper and 40% nickel). The two wires are spot welded together to form secure junctions. The copper wire is cut to allow for the insertion of a microvoltmeter or chart recorder calibrated in degrees Celsius, Figure 4.1. One of the junctions is held at a constant temperature. This could be 0 degrees Celsius by placing the junction in a thermos flask of melting ice or in a metal block whose temperature is controlled electronically at a known value. When a temperature difference exists between the junctions the thermocouple generates a thermal electromotive force. This amounts to 40 microvolts per degree centigrade difference between the junctions for a copper-constantan combination. Thus, for the 'cold' junction at 0 degrees Celsius and the 'hot'

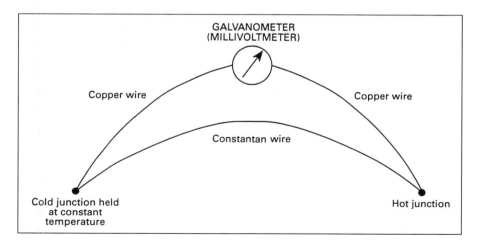

Figure 4.1 Schematic diagram of a thermocouple circuit.

junction at 37 degrees Celsius the output from the thermocouple amounts to 1.48 millivolts which can easily be handled by a potentiometric type chart recorder.

Thermocouples offer the advantage of reproducible calibrations and it is easy to make a set of thermocouples from two reels of wire. The 'hot junction' can be small, depending on the diameter chosen for the wires and can be inserted into the lumen of a hypodermic needle for taking temperatures in muscle.

4.7 Cleaning of clinical thermometers

Clarke (1992) asked doctors how they cleaned thermometers after use. The majority of users either rinsed the device under a tap with or without soap (38%) or used an alcohol swab (38%), 12% soaked the device in sodium hypochlorite solution (Milton), 5% washed it with chlorhexidene (Hibitane), 1% used the thermometer with an external disposable sheath and 6% did not clean the thermometer.

4.8 Variations in the body temperature of infants at night

There is increasing evidence that overheating is a contributing factor for some cot deaths (Brown, P. J., Dove, R. A., Tuffnell, C. S. and Ford R. P. K. (1992) 'Oscillations of body temperature at night', *Archives of Diseases of Childhood*, **67**, 1255–8. It has been suggested that thermoregulation in infants is closely connected to their respiratory control. Brown *et al.* (1992) used semiconductor temperature sensors rather than thermistors to monitor rectal temperature 5 cm from the anal margin and skin temperature from the forehead, axilla, wrist, abdomen, shin and foot. Each temperature channel was sampled once per second and the readings stored in a computer for subsequent analysis. Recording time overnight was at least 12 hours. Sleep state, feeds, nappy changes and other behaviour were recorded on a diary sheet and also by continuous video recording. Software was written to produce a spectral analysis of the data with peaks corresponding with dominant oscillations. Oscillations which varied in amplitude by more than 0.1 degrees Celsius were measured for the length of periods from peak to peak and the average period calculated. The variation in rectal temperature over a single night was 0.4 to 0.7 degrees Celsius in infants less than eight weeks old but in those more than 12 weeks old it could be as much as 1.5 degrees Celsius.

In infants less than four weeks old the axillary temperature reflected the rectal temperature fairly well, but in older infants this was not so. The wrist, shin and foot temperatures showed opposite trends to the rectal temperatures, with a rapid increase of several degrees over the first hour after falling asleep, and a rapid decrease when waking for a feed or nappy change. The forehead temperature followed neither the rectal nor the 'peripheral' pattern.

In addition to these sleep-wake patterns there was a small amplitude oscillation of rectal temperature in 24 of the 30 continuous recordings. The amplitude of the oscillation was 0.2 to 0.3 degrees Celsius and the period was about 60 minutes. This study by Brown et al. (1992) confirms the complexity of the factors which affect body temperatures. Apart from the need for accurate temperature measurements at a variety of body sites, the interpretation of multiple temperature measurements needs considerable care. A further paper dealing with night-time temperature rhythms in infants is that of Lodemore, M. R., Peterson, S. A. and Wailoo, M. P. (1992) 'Factors affecting the development of night-time temperature rhythms', *Archives of Diseases of Childhood*, **67**, 1259–61.

4.9 Temperature monitoring in relation to the Sudden Infant Death Syndrome

An increased body temperature, possibly due to an excess of clothing, has been postulated as a factor conducive to the Sudden Infant Death Syndrome (SIDS). One approach to monitoring infants thought to be at risk is to place an insulated temperature sensor against the baby's skin and held in place by the nappy band. A soft cable is taken out from beneath the nappy on the outside of the baby's leg. It connects with a battery-powered alarm unit located at the foot of the cot and inaccessible to the baby's head and limbs. The alarm is activated when the temperature attains 37.5 degrees Celsius at which the infant is believed to be in possible distress.

4.10 Thermal dilution method for the measurement of cardiac output

Cardiac output is defined as the volume of blood in litres pumped per minute by the heart. The accurate recording of the temperature of arterial blood occurs with the thermal dilution method for estimating cardiac output. Although invasive, the method is widely used in major intensive care units and is based on recording the change in temperature with time produced in a bolus of cool saline or 5% dextrose in sterile water as the bolus passes a thermistor blood-temperature sensor.

Adequate mixing of the volume (5 or 10 ml) of saline previously cooled to a known temperature, perhaps 0.5 degrees Celsius, and arterial blood can be obtained by interposing one cardiac chamber between the sites of detection and injection. Injection may be into the right atrium and subsequent detection in the pulmonary artery, with two separate catheters passed via vessels in the neck. Alternatively, a double lumen catheter (6 or 7 French gauge) having a thermistor at its tip can be positioned with its tip in the pulmonary artery and the opening of the injection lumen situated in the right atrium. The catheter also allows for continuous monitoring of pressure in the right atrium, pulmonary artery and pulmonary capillaries and the withdrawal of blood from the pulmonary artery for oxygen measurements. The catheter has an inflatable balloon at its tip so that it is flow directed. The thermistor is embedded in the catheter wall just proximal to the balloon and the time constant for temperature recording is about one second. The second lumen is located 30 cm behind the tip to ensure that with the tip in the pulmonary artery the opening lies in the right atrium. The other lumen opens at the tip of the catheter. A 5 French gauge version is available for paediatric studies. The catheter is specially designed to minimize the transfer of heat from the warm arterial blood to the cool saline as this is rapidly injected in less than four seconds. Prior to the injection, the calibrated thermistor records the blood temperature, typically 37 degrees Celsius. As the bolus of saline passes by, the recorded temperature falls, perhaps to 36.8 degrees and then rises back to 37 degrees over a period of several seconds. A plot of the fall in blood temperature and the subsequent rise against time is known as a thermal dilution curve, Figure 4.2. From a knowledge of the volume of the injectate, the initial temperature of the injectate, the initial blood temperature and the area under the dilution curve, a microprocessor can easily calculate the cardiac output.

The cardiac output in 1 per minute is given by:

cardiac output $= Vi \times (Tb - Ti) \times K \times Ct/A$, where

Vi = injectate volume in litres
Tb = blood temperature in degrees Celsius
Ti = temperature of injectate at entry to blood stream in degrees Celsius
K = A factor relating the specific heat and density of blood and water and the conversion of seconds to minutes $= 1.08$
     where $1.08 =$ (density $\times$ specific heat) injectate/(density $\times$ specific heat) blood
A = the area of the thermodilution curve in seconds $\times$ degrees Celsius
Ct = catheter loss factor

Figure 4.2 Thermodilution curve.

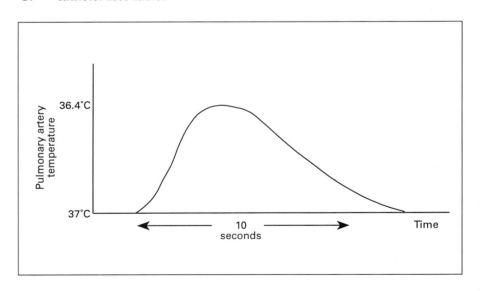

In practice if the injectate at 0.5 degrees Celsius has warmed up to 7 degrees on leaving the catheter the expected value of (Tb-Ti) is (37-0.5) = 36.5 degrees whereas the actual value is (37-7) = 30 degrees so that Ct = 30/36.5 = 0.82. As an example suppose that A = 3 degrees × seconds, then cardiac output = 1.08 × 0.82 × 60 × 0.01 × 36.5 /3 = 6.5 litres per minute. The various factors involved are input to a cardiac-output computer which then measures the area under the thermodilution curve and calculates the cardiac output.

For an adult having a normal heart and at rest, the cardiac output is likely to be about 5 litres per minute. For a heart rate of 70 beats per minute, the volume of blood pumped per beat, the stroke volume, is 5000/70 = 71.4 ml. The cardiac output and the stroke volume can each be normalized to give the cardiac index and the stroke index respectively by dividing by the body surface area in square metres. The cool injectate is innocuous and repeated cardiac output determinations can be made without harm to the patient. The thermodilution methods yield an average cardiac output over several successive beats and the value could be affected by the presence of ectopic beats.

Thermal dilution is often used as a 'standard' method against which to compare other non-invasive methods such as Doppler shift ultrasound and electrical impedance which operate on a beat-by-beat basis, e.g. Castor, G., Helms, J., Niedermark, I., Molter, G., Motsch, J. and Altmeyer, P. (1991) 'Influence of the ventilatory cycle on cardiac output determination during mechanical ventilation. A comparison of non-invasive electrical bioimpedance with standard thermodilution method', *American Journal of Noninvasive Cardiology*, **5**, 57–61; and Mellander, M., Sabel, K. G., Caidahl, K., Solymar, L. and Eriksson, B. (1987) 'Doppler determination of cardiac output in infants and children: comparison with simultaneous thermodilution' *Pediatric Cardiology*, **8**, 241–6.

5 Respiratory function tests

5.1 Introduction

The full range of respiratory function tests available in a modern acute hospital is considerable and in some cases makes use of bulky spirometer systems, a body plethysmograph and sensitive gas analysers such as a mass spectrometer. Tests available for use with conscious and cooperative patients can include: respiratory volumes and flow rates under normal breathing and forced conditions, airways resistance and lung-diffusing capacity. Intensive care situations blood-gas and pH measurements will be available but other tests will be limited to compact equipment such as a dry spirometer, peak flowmeter, respirometer and pneumotachograph which can be used with patients either in bed or sitting up not far away.

5.2 The dry spirometer

The forced vital capacity of a patient is the maximal volume of gas which can be expelled from the lungs by a forceful effort following a maximal inspiration. It has the following sub-divisions: inspiratory reserve volume (the maximum amount of gas which can be inspired from the end-inspiratory level), expiratory reserve volume (the maximum volume of gas which can be expired from the end-expiratory level) and tidal volume (the volume of gas inspired or expired during each respiratory cycle). The minute volume is the volume of gas respired over a period of one minute. All these variables can be measured on a patient who can cooperate by means of a simple volume recorder such as a dry spirometer. The residual volume is the volume of gas remaining in the lungs after a maximal forced expiration. The functional residual capacity is the sum of the expiratory reserve volume and the residual volume. The inspiratory capacity is the sum of the tidal volume and the inspiratory reserve volume. The total lung capacity is the sum of the vital capacity and the residual volume, Figure 5.1.

Figure 5.1 The relationship of pulmonary volumes and capacities during normal respiration and with a maximum inspiration and expiration.

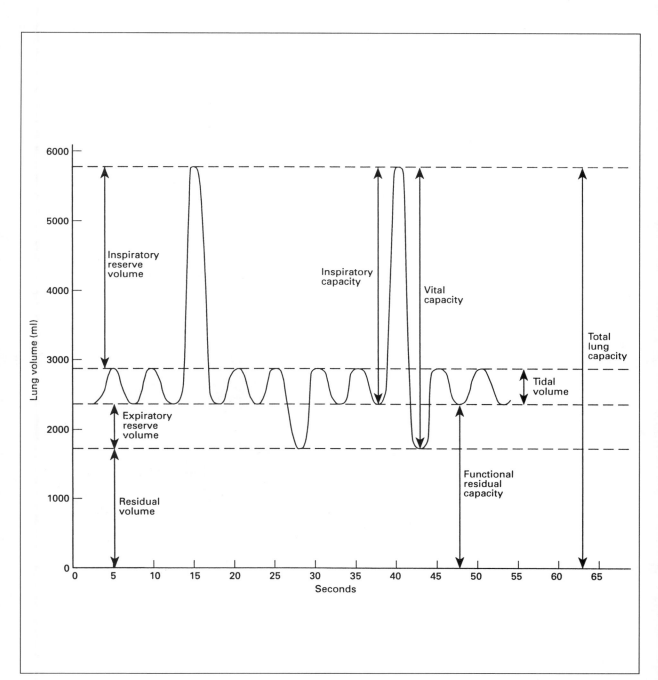

For intensive care situations a suitable equipment is a dry wedge bellows spirometer which has a low resistance to airflow, Figure 5.2. Basically, it comprises a gas holder into which the patient exhales, while wearing a noseclip, via a disposable mouthpiece at the end of the flexible inlet tube. As the bellows expands while taking up the expired gas volume, it causes a pen to move across a paper chart scaled in litres for the vertical axis and in seconds (0 to 6) on the horizontal axis. After taking a maximal inspiration, the patient is encouraged to exhale at his maximum rate. The chart deflection can be read off in terms of forced vital capacity, forced expiratory volume achieved at the end of one second, forced expiratory flow rate in litres per second between definite points such as expired volumes of 0.2 and 1.2 litres and the forced mid-expiratory flow time. The capacity of such a dry spirometer is approximately 8 litres. Lung volumes and expiratory flow rates are quoted in litres BTPS (Body Temperature and Pressure Saturated at body temperature with water vapour). The values will actually be measured in a room under ambient conditions ATPS (Ambient Temperature and Pressure Saturated). A conversion factor must be applied to convert values measured under ATPS conditions to those which correspond with BTPS conditions.

As an example, a patient's minute volume is measured as 6 litres under ATPS conditions (laboratory temperature 20 degrees Celsius; barometric pressure 760 mmHg; saturated water-vapour pressure 18 mmHg at 20

Figure 5.2 Vitalograph dry wedge spirometer. (Courtesy Vitalograph Ltd.)

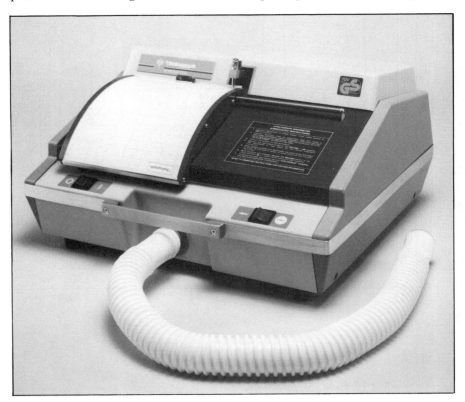

degrees and 47 mmHg at 37 degrees). Referred to BTPS conditions the minute volume becomes 6.61 litres. The calculation uses the fact that for a given mass of gas (Pressure $\times$ Volume)/Absolute Temperature $=$ a constant value. The Absolute Temperature is found by adding 273 to the temperature in degrees Celsius. Thus $(760\text{-}18) \times 6/(273+20) = (760–37) \times V/(273 + 37)$ and $V = 6.61$ litres.

5.3 The peak flowmeter

This is a hand-held device to which can be fitted a disposable cardboard mouthpiece or a plastic mouthpiece which can be washed and sterilized. In one version, the patient makes a forced expiration into the meter which causes a closely fitting vane to sweep round a cylindrical cavity, the vane not touching the sides of the cavity. A spiral spring is attached to one end of the spindle about which the vane rotates. A pointer attached to the other end of the spindle counterbalances the vane and indicates its position on a circular scale calibrated over the range 50 to 1000 litres per minute. As the flow of expired air from the patient rotates the vane against the tension of the spring, the movement of the vane uncovers an increasing aperture of an annular orifice running round the periphery of the circular chamber. Air can escape from the chamber via the orifice. When the area of the orifice uncovered by the vane is just sufficient to produce a chamber pressure in front of the vane which will counterbalance the force exerted by the spring, the vane will come to rest with a deflection which is dependent upon the peak flow rate. The spring tension increases with deflection reducing the vane's deflection for high flow rates relative to those for low flow rates. A ratchet is arranged to hold the vane at the position of maximum deflection until it is manually released to enable the peak flow rate to be read off from the scale. The average reading is taken from three attempts.

5.4 The turbine respirometer

This widely encountered device is based on a miniature air turbine designed to have a rotor with a very low inertia. In the original mechanical versions, the rotations of the twin-blade rotor were counted with a watch-type gear train driving hands sweeping over a dial scaled in litres, (Wright, B. M. A. (1955) 'Respiratory anemometer', *Journal of Physiology*, **127**, 25P).

The turbine arrangement is self-rectifying and only records the volume of gas which passes through the respirometer in the forward direction with each expiration. Gas entering the respirometer emerges from a series of fixed tangential slots to strike the rotor in such a fashion that the rotor responds only to gas flow in the forward direction and no valves are required. The turbine respirometer must be located in the breathing circuit in such a position that expired water vapour cannot collect in the turbine chamber as this would affect the calibration.

The ratio of the gas volume recorded to that actually passing through the device is flow-rate dependent because the slip of gas past the rotor will be greater at the higher flow rates resulting in a non-linear calibration (Nunn, J. F. and Ezi-Ashi, T. I. (1962) 'The accuracy of the respirometer and ventigrator', *British Journal of Anaesthesia*, **34**, 422–4). This mechanical system is compact and lightweight, but can be damaged by being inadvertently dropped. The problem then is that the respirometer still appears to function but its reading may be inaccurate. Later versions of respirometer have the mechanical gear train replaced with a beam of light which is interrupted periodically by the turbine blades as they rotate. The resulting pulses of light fall on to a photocell giving rise to a train of electrical pulses which are then counted and totalled over a minute and displayed in terms of scales covering the ranges 0.2 to 15 and 4 to 30 litres per minute on a panel meter or digital display.

An alternative arrangement uses a magnetic pick-up to detect the rotation of the turbine's rotor and generates two equal square wave electrical pulses per revolution of the rotor, the pulse repetition frequency being 80 Hz at 16 litres per minute continuous gas flow. The turbine flow head, Figure 5.3, can be sterilized by autoclaving at temperatures up to 136 degrees Celsius or with ethylene oxide. The coupling of the rotor via a magnetic field through the wall of the casing to the detecting sensor isolates oxygen and anaesthetic vapours from the pulse-counting circuitry. The maximum safe flow rate is 300 litres per minute and the resistance to respiration is proportional to the square of the volume flow rate and does not exceed 2 cm of water at 100 litres per minute. The minimum operating flowrate is approximately two litres per minute. A selector switch on the

Figure 5.3 Magtrak turbine gas-flow sensor. (Courtesy Ferraris Development and Engineering Company Ltd.)

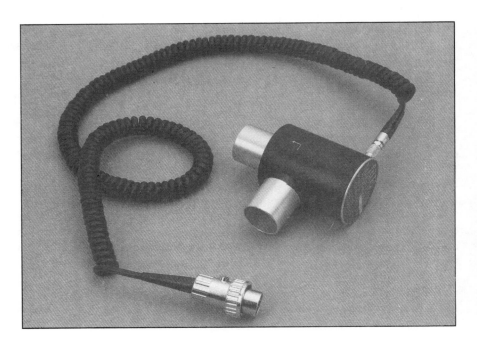

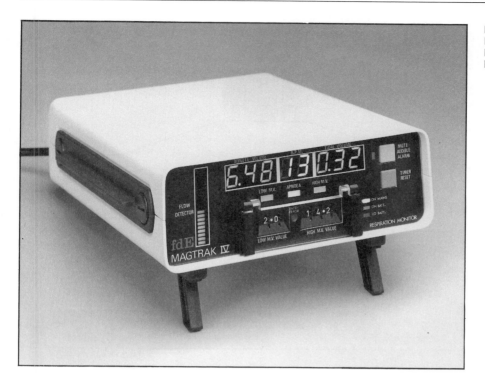

Figure 5.4 Magtrak IV Respiratory Monitor. (Courtesy Ferraris Development and Engineering Company Ltd.)

control unit provides a choice of minute volume, tidal volume or respiratory rate to be displayed, Figure 5.4. Both audible and visible alarms are activated if gas flow has not been detected for 15 seconds. Battery back-up is provided for use when mains power is not available.

5.5 The pneumotachograph

Basically, a pneumotachograph consists of an arrangement such as a fine mesh wire gauze operating as a low resistance to gas flow. The design is such that the pressure drop developed across the gauze is directly proportional to the volume flow rate over a stated volume flow range. Typically, the resistance to gas flow might be a sheet of 400 mesh wire gauze supported around the periphery at the centre of a double cone-shaped metal flow head. By means of annular pressure pick-up channels located close to each side of the gauze the pressure drop developed across the gauze when gas is flowing is led off via a pair of rubber or plastic tubes connecting to each input of a sensitive differential pressure transducer, Figure 5.5. In the case of a relatively small pneumotachograph head the maximum flow rate of 180 litres per minute would generate a pressure drop of approximately 6 mm of water.

Using a suitable source of gas-flow rates, such as a good quality vacuum cleaner in conjunction with a calibrated gas flowmeter, the electrical output signal from the pressure transducer can be displayed on a chart

Figure 5.5 Cross-section of a
wire-gauge-type pneumotachograph head.

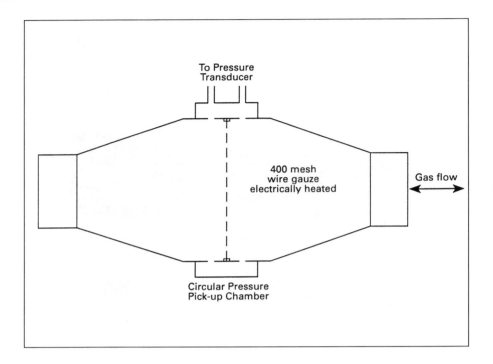

Figure 5.5 Cross-section of a wire-gauge-type pneumotachograph head.

recorder and calibrated in litres per minute using a standard gas flowmeter. This arrangement is useful for recording breathing waveforms. It will show both forward and reverse flow patterns. By integrating the output from the pneumotachograph the volume flow tracing is transformed into a tidal volume tracing scaled in terms of millilitres, and by integrating over a minute and then resetting to zero a minute volume tracing can be obtained. Any inequality in the calibration for forward and reverse flow will produce a shift in the baseline of the chart-recorder tracing and a regular resetting to zero may be necessary. To prevent condensation of water vapour from expired air on the gauze it is usual to heat the gauze by passing an electrical current through it from a low voltage supply. When using a pneumotachograph head with rapidly changing gas-flow waveforms, such as those produced by some types of automatic lung ventilator, it is important to securely anchor the tubes leading to the pressure transducer and to equalize the pneumatic capacities of the tubes in order to minimize artifact deflections occurring on the flow record. These arise when the pressure pulse does not arrive simultaneously at each side of the pressure transducer's diaphragm.

5.6 Expected values

Formulae exist to predict 'normal' values for a number of respiratory function tests where the predicted values are based upon variables such as the patient's body surface area, height, weight and age. For example: for males vital capacity = $(27.63 - (0.112 \times age)) \times$ height in cm. Thus for a 20-year-old man 6 feet (183 cm) tall, the vital capacity is 4610 ml. Charts are available showing the variation of peak expiratory flowrate with age for men and for women and nomograms relating height and age to vital capacity, peak expiratory flowrate, residual volume and forced expiratory volume after one second of expiration. As ever, care must be taken in interpreting the measured and predicted values in the context of the patient's clinical condition.

5.7 Gas and vapour analysers

In some intensive care situations such as major surgery under general anaesthesia it is important to monitor on a regular basis variables such as the inspired oxygen concentration (typically with a fuel cell type of oxygen monitor), end-tidal and inspiratory carbon dioxide levels (using infra-red gas analysis) and the patient's percentage oxygen saturation (by means of a pulse oximeter). Infra-red gas analysis is also applicable to the monitoring of the concentrations in an anaesthetic circuit of carbon dioxide, nitrous oxide and the volatile anaesthetic agents halothane, enflurane and isoflurane, Figure 5.6 (a). Gas and vapour monitor cabinets can be mounted on anaesthetic machines to allow monitoring of these gas and vapour concentrations together with tidal and minute volume and respiratory rate – all with associated alarm facilites (Figure 5.6 (b)).

Carbon dioxide absorbs infra-red radiation strongly at a wavelength of 4.25 micrometres and nitrous oxide at 4.49 micrometres as examples. A heated metal spiral provides a broadband source of infra-red radiation. This is directed at a motor-driven rotating disk which carries a series of optical filters to select wavelengths to act as a reference where there is no absorption and wavelengths which are specific to the absorption characteristics of the particular gases and vapours. Pulses of light of the selected wavelengths produced by the rotating disk are passed through a sample

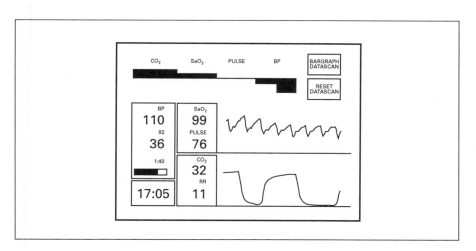

Figure 5.6 (a) Monitor screen display showing the output signal from a pulse oximeter indicating a heart rate of 76 beats per minute and oxygen saturation of 99% together with the output signal from an infra-red non-dispersive gas analyser indicating an end-tidal carbon dioxide partial pressure of 32 mm Hg at a respiratory rate of 11 breaths per minute. Clock time and blood pressures are also displayed. (Courtesy North American Drager.)

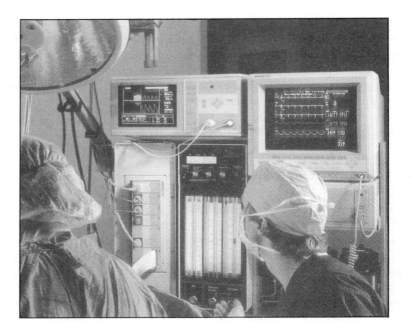

cell fitted with windows of a material which will transmit the infra-red wavelengths. A pump continuously sucks a small sample of the gas mixture to be analysed through the sample cell. In the cell the reference beam passes through almost unchanged, whereas the intensity of the other wavelengths will be diminished by absorption if the particular gas or vapour concerned is present in the sample mixture.

The emergent infra-red beam falls on an indium antimonide or other suitable infra-red detector. The ratios of the detector signals for the reference wavelength and each gas or vapour wavelength are calibrated in terms of the concentration in the mixture of each component. The rotating disk with its set of optical filters interrupts or 'chops' the infra-red radiation and the amplifier used with the solid-state infra-red detector is tuned to this chopping frequency to reduce the influence of noise or random signals.

Typical ranges might be carbon dioxide 0 to 10.5% by volume, nitrous oxide 0 to 100%, halothane 0 to 8.5%, enflurane 0 to 8.5% and isoflurane 0 to 8.5%. With a flowrate through the analyser of 200 ml per minute, the response time (10% to 90%) for carbon dioxide and nitrous oxide is 200 milliseconds and for the volatile agents 400 milliseconds. With the appropriate make of anaesthetic vaporizer the gas and vapour analyser is automatically signalled when one of the volatile agent vaporizers is turned ON. An apnoea alarm is obtained by monitoring for an absence of respiratory fluctuations in the carbon dioxide level. If a portable, relatively low cost and accuracy carbon dioxide analyser is available it can be used in emergency care situations to check that an endotracheal tube has been passed into the trachea rather than the oesophagus.

5.8 Applications of respiratory function tests

Tests involving the dry spirometer and peak flow meter require a conscious and cooperative patient capable of producing a maximal inspiration and expiration. Similarly, the evaluation of bronchodilator therapy requires the measurement of peak flow rates. The routine measurement of minute and tidal volumes and gas and anaesthetic concentrations are important in the management of anaesthetized and ventilated patients and those recovering from thoracic surgery and drug overdoses.

5.9 Respiratory rate monitors

A requirement often arises to monitor respiration rate e.g. for gating the monitoring of other variables or synchronizing imaging devices to a particular phase of respiration. A thermistor probe can be placed beneath a nostril to detect the cyclic changes of respired air temperature, or a two-electrode impedance system operating at 25 kHz can be used to monitor changes in the patient's thoracic electrical impedance occurring with respiration. The impedance of an adult thorax measured with a pair of 10 cm diameter silver disk electrodes is typically 200 ohms and changes by approximately 2.5 ohms per litre tidal volume.

The impedance technique with an elasticated belt electrode is also used for the respiration monitoring of babies suspected of being vulnerable to the Sudden Infant Death Syndrome (SIDS). The risk factors for SIDS are discussed by: Mitchell et al. (1993) 'Ethnic differences in mortality from sudden infant death syndrome in New Zealand', *British Medical Journal*, **306**, 13–16; and by Gantley, M., Davies, D. P. and Murcott, A. (1993) 'Sudden infant death syndrome: links with infant care practices', *British Medical Journal*, **306**, 16–20. Other approaches to the detection of apnoea in infants have involved the use of a segmented air-filled mattress with the segments connected by tubes arranged to puff air over a thermistor when respiratory movements were present and detection of the Doppler frequency shift when a beam of 10 GHz microwave radiation was reflected from the baby's moving chest.

6 Electrophysiological measurements

6.1 Introduction

As the name suggests, electrophysiological measurements are concerned with the measurement, and usually recording, of the electrical activity associated with particular physiological functions such as the beating of the heart – the electrocardiogram (ECG). In practice, electrical activity may be detected from more than one physiological function, e.g. the waveform of the ECG may be influenced (modulated) by the slower waveform due to respiration producing motion of the thorax. It may be necessary to use a hardware or software filter to separate one waveform from another. A classic case arises with the interaction of the maternal ECG with the foetal ECG.

The ECG is normally a periodic waveform developing with each set of contractions and relaxations of the atria and ventricles during each cardiac cycle. Experienced observers of the ECG can distinguish between those portions of the waveform associated with the atria and the ventricles. The shape of the ECG waveform depends not only on the condition of the heart but also on the positioning of the electrodes used to pick up the ECG. When recording an ECG it is important to place the electrodes at internationally standardized positions to allow intercomparisons between patients and for a particular patient at different times. A standard amplitude signal (usually one millivolt) must also be recorded as a calibration to allow determination of the amplitude of the ECG. It is also important to reduce artifacts which might appear on the recording by using good quality, electrically stable, electrodes securely affixed to the skin. It must be remembered that the practical recording of electrophysiological signals from seriously ill patients can present challenges markedly different from the situation found when recording from fit, young volunteers in the laboratory.

While the ECG is likely to be the most commonly measured electrophysiological signal in intensive care situations, the electroencephalogram (EEG) is recorded from electrodes attached to the scalp as a check on the adequacy of cerebral function during major surgery and possibly during the assessment of 'brain death'. Unlike the regularly repeating rhythms of the ECG, the EEG is much more random in nature and about one tenth the amplitude of a normal ECG. For interpretation, the EEG is divided into several frequency bands and the content of these, together wih the nature of the activity, is taken into account by a clinical neurophysiologist. The electrical activity of muscles also generates an electrophysiological signal: the electromyogram (EMG). For a striated muscle the electrical activity produced consists of a series of short duration spikes whose activity markedly increases when the muscle contracts. The frequency content of the EMG extends out to several hundred hertz in contrast to that of a diagnostic quality ECG which will not exceed 100 Hz. The EMG of a smooth muscle such as the gut or bladder is more like that of an EEG and the EMG of the gut will exhibit marked peristaltic activity: Chen, J., McCallum, R. W. and Richards, R. (1993) 'Frequency components of the electrogastrogram and their correlations with gastrointestinal contractions in humans', *Medical and Biological Engineering and Computing*, **31**, 60–7.

Another type of electrophysiological measurement is the recording of evoked responses to given stimuli. Work has currently focused on elements of the EEG, for example, giving an auditory stimulus and recording the response from bi-polar leads with electrodes positioned on the scalp over the auditory centres of the brain.

6.2 Generation of the electrocardiogram

The body and its fluids represents a conductor of electricity inside which the heart, acting both as an electrical generator and a pump for blood, gives rise to a time varying electric field which appears on the skin as a series of varying potentials which can be picked up by suitably positioned recording electrodes. The electrical activity initiates the mechanical contraction of the ventricles. By feeding the signals into an ECG amplifier and then to a suitable display, the time rate of change of the potentials can be shown in the form of the ECG waveform. The combination of at least two electrodes attached to the patient at specific locations is known as an ECG lead.

The simplest ECG leads are known as the Einthoven Leads, I, II and III after the pioneer of electrocardiography Einthoven. Electrodes are placed on the patient's left and right wrists and left ankle. Lead I is recorded between the left and right wrists, Lead II between the right wrist and left ankle and Lead III between the left wrist and left ankle, Figure 6.1. A normal set of Lead I, II and III ECGs is illustrated in Figure 6.2 which shows that the three waveforms are markedly different.

Considering the Lead I tracing in more detail, Figure 6.3, the large positive spike is the R-wave which is synchronous with the contracting of the ventricles. If it commences with an initial negative wave this is called the Q-wave and if it finishes with a negative wave this is called the S-wave

Figure 6.1 Standard Electrocardiogram Leads I, II and III. (By courtesy of Hewlett Packard Ltd.)

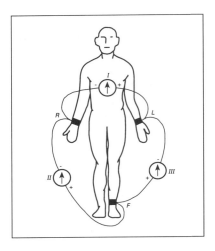

Figure 6.2 Normal set of Lead I, II and III ECGs produced on 12-lead ECG machine. (By courtesy of Hewlett Packard Ltd.)

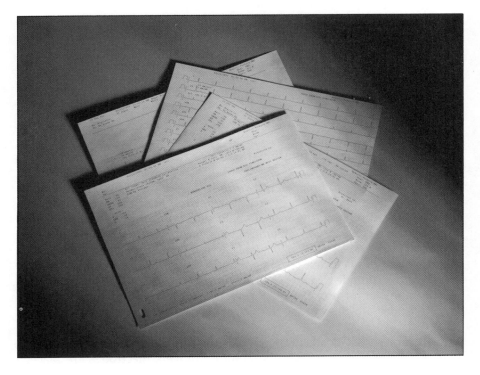

so that the complete R-wave from beginning to end is also known as the QRS complex. Its normal duration is 0.05 to 0.10 seconds. The preceding wave is the P-wave which is generated by the contraction of the atria. Its normal duration does not exceed 0.11 seconds. After the QRS complex occurs the T-wave which is generated by the resetting of the ventricles ready for their next contraction.

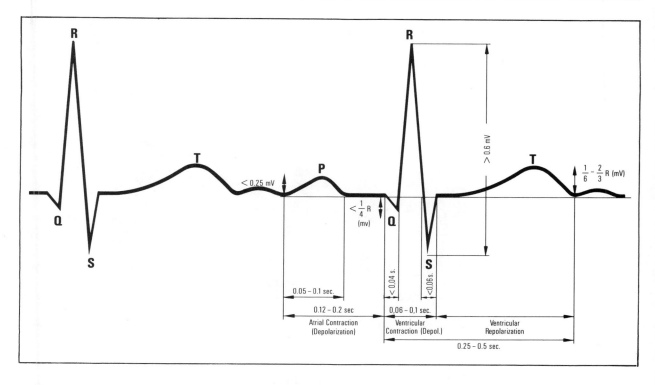

Figure 6.3 One cardiac cycle of a Lead I ECG. (By courtesy of Hewlett Packard Ltd.)

Between the P-wave and the QRS complex lies the P-R segment which is normally lying close to the baseline (isoelectric line). Its normal duration is 0.1 to 0.2 seconds and depends on the heart rate. The S-T segment lies between the end of the QRS complex and the start of the T-wave. It is normally close to the baseline but significant elevation or depression of the S-T segment from the baseline may have a diagnostic significance, e.g. S-T segment depression may be an indicator of myocardial ischaemia having occurred.

In addition to Leads I, II and III a set of six smaller chest electrodes can be placed at specific and standard positions on the patient's chest. For a full diagnostic ECG as used in a cardiology clinic a selector switch is used to select 12 various combinations of limb and chest electrodes to produce a 12-lead ECG. For speed and convenience the 12 tracings may be recorded as four sets of three waveforms on an automatic 3-channel ECG recorder.

The requirements for an ECG in intensive care situations may be simpler and disposable chest electrodes may be used to simulate Leads I, II and III. The positioning and type of electrode is aimed at reducing artifacts due to patient movement. A good R-wave may be required to trigger the circuitry of a heart-rate recorder. Software templates of a particular patient's ECG are used in modern patient monitors to maximize the reliability of heart-rate recording and the reduction of false alarms.

Rather than monitor just the ECG, in some situations it is necessary to monitor real-time displays of a group of cardiac functions, as seen in Figure 6.4.

Figure 6.4 Monitor showing a
group of cardiac functions. (By
courtesy of Hewlett Packard Ltd.)

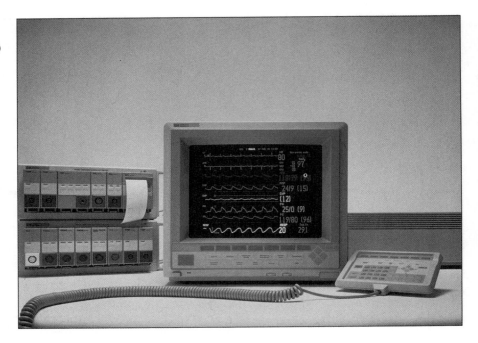

Figure 6.4 Monitor showing a group of cardiac functions. (By courtesy of Hewlett Packard Ltd.)

6.3 The ambulatory monitoring of ECGs

Cardiac problems in a patient may only present when the patient is active, for example climbing stairs, or getting up in the night to urinate. The requirement for the ECG in mobile patients initially led to the development of small, battery-powered tape recorders which could be carried by the patients and which could record several hours of ECG. In the USA this technique became known as Holter recording after its developer. The electromechanical tape recorder has now been replaced with a solid-state memory. In one model there are two recording channels each with a 0.05 to 25 Hz (–3 dB) bandwidth. The memory is 11.5 megabytes which store 48 hours of single-channel or 24 hours of two-channel ECGs. The recorder is powered by 6 alkaline batteries and weighs approximately 1 kg. A high speed playback system is available which can be programmed to pick up irregularities in the ECG. Versions of solid-state recorders are available to record the arterial blood pressure and EEG from ambulatory patients.

An alternative approach utilizes radiotelemetry where the patient carries a small radio transmitter which transmits the physiological signals via a radio link back to a central station. This technique is useful for patients in an intermediate care ward where monitoring is still necessary, but the patient is not confined to bed. The system must be designed to have an adequate range of transmission in relation to the siting of the receiving aerial. A loss of signal, perhaps due to a patient being behind a steel girder, must not be confused with asystole.

6.4 The measurement of electrophysiological signals

A typical muscle cell at rest exists in a polarized state, the electrical potential of the cell being negative by about 100 millivolts relative to the potential existing at the cell's surface. This steady potential difference is known as the membrane potential. It is maintained by means of a sodium-pump mechanism which is an active process in the living cell serving to exclude sodium ions from the cell's interior. A transient increase in the permeability of the cell's membrane to sodium ions can occur, causing the cell to depolarize and the sign of the potential difference across the membrane reverses, the interior of the cell now being approximately 25 millivolts higher (positive) with respect to the cell's surface. Depolarization is shortly followed by contraction of the cell. After depolarization the cell more slowly repolarizes and returns to its resting state. This transient change in potential difference of the interior of the cell from −100 mV to +25 mV is known as an action potential.

The tissues responsible for the initiation and conduction of the wave of action potentials responsible for each heart beat are found at the sino-atrial node, the atrial-ventricular node and the Bundle of His. Of critical importance to the maintenance of the heartbeat are two differences from normal muscle contraction: the transmembrane potentials of these specialized tissues are less negative, at around −70 mV; and they 'leak' sodium ions, allowing the automatic triggering of action potentials, normally at a rate of about 70 times per minute.

For patients with a basically low heart rate (bradycardia) it may be necessary to fit them with an implanted electronic cardiac pacemaker. This consists of a circuit which is hermetically sealed within a metal enclosure covered with a biologically inert substance such as silicone rubber in order to prevent rejection by the body. The circuit is powered by a lithium battery having a life of several years and is planted in a subcutaneous pocket in the axilla. It feeds electrical pulses, typically at a rate of 70 per minute, via a flexible metal pacing lead which has a barbed tip embedded in the apex of the right ventricle. The regular series of pulses 'pace' the heart at the predetermined rate in the simplest type of electronic pacemaker. More sophisticated versions can respond to increases in rate of the heart's natural pacemaker if this is functioning, but a defect exists in the conduction pathways leading from it.

Patients fitted with electronic pacemakers can be at risk from the influence of surgical diathermy, magnetic fields in excess of 5 gauss (important in magnetic resonance imaging (MRI)) or leakage currents from patient monitors. Strict safety precautions must be observed with such patients in any of these situations. Implanted cardiac pacemakers are designed to cater for patients with chronic conditions.

External cardiac pacing is an acute procedure using a battery-powered cardiac pacemaker unit situated outside the patient's body. The pacemaker is connected to a temporary cardiac-pacing catheter which is brought out percutaneously. Patients having an externalized pacing catheter are also at considerable electrical risk. As discussed in Chapter 15, currents in excess of 100 microamperes at mains frequency can be potentially lethal. Alternatively, in an emergency, pacing can be accomplished via metal gauze or plate electrodes used with conducting electrode gel and placed over the manubrium and the left axilla just lateral to the apex beat.

Some types of defibrillator can be provided with a cardiac pacemaker for external pacing. A constant current circuit is used with the pacing current being adjustable in the range 30 mA to 200 mA with a pulse width of 20 ms and a pacing rate variable between 40 to 180 pulses per minute. The patient may need to be anaesthetized to overcome pain arising from the muscular contractions.

For internal pacing via a pacing lead embedded in the apex of the right ventricle a maximum pulse amplitude of 15 V is required compared with 150 V for external pacing. The temporary pacing catheter may be positioned under direct visual control by means of a mobile X-ray image intensifier unit designed for bedside use. Alternatively, a 3 or 5 French balloon float catheter may be used having two metal electrodes situated at its distal tip and separated by a 1 cm long inflatable balloon. The pacing rate is initially set to be greater than the spontaneous heart rate and the stimulating current per pulse is gradually reduced until the pacemaker loses control of the heart. The current is then increased to perhaps double the value at which control was lost.

Patients having an externalized pacing catheter are also electrically at considerable risk. Whenever the pacemaker terminals are handled, the operator should wear surgical rubber gloves as insulation and no other object (e.g. bedframe, bedside lamp or patient monitor) should be touched at the same time. It is vital that leakage currents are prevented from flowing into the heart via the pacing catheter.

The sino-atrial node is situated in the right atrium and covers an area of approximately 2 mm × 20 mm. It is supplied with many nerve fibres and has its own rich blood supply. The muscle cells of the sino-atrial node are one-third the size of normal cardiac muscle cells and fusiform in shape. In terms of a strip of muscle fibre, the process of depolarization generates a wave of electrical activity which spreads along adjacent cells, causing them to contract. This electrical activity reaches the atrial-ventricular node 0.04 seconds after leaving the sino-atrial node. The nerve fibres of the atrial-ventricular node have a small diameter, which prevents rapid conduction of the wave of depolarization, and the conduction velocity is about 0.05 metres per second. The speed of conduction increases to 0.1 metres per second after leaving the atrial-ventricular node, as the size of the cardiac muscle cells increases. Thus, the spontaneous electrical activity appearing in the sino-atrial node passes through the atrial-ventricular node, then passes forward and downwards into the inter-ventricular septum (Bundle of His), splits into the two bundle branches serving the right and left ventricles. These give off many fine branches which form a reticulated layer just beneath the endocardium – the Purkinje tissue. Cardiac muscle cells here are very large, and yield a high conduction velocity of between 1.5 and 2.5 metres per second. As a result, the ventricles contract sharply during the systolic phase of the cardiac cycle.

The electrical activity of the beating heart is transmitted through the body tissues to the skin where it can be picked up by suitably positioned recording electrodes. The normal rhythmic coordinated beating of the heart is known as sinus rhythm, with the atria and ventricles contracting in an efficient cycle to pump blood around the body.

The sino-atrial node is known as the pacemaker because it is the centre which initiates the wave of depolarization leading to the heartbeat. On occasion, the heartbeat can originate from the other centres of automatic muscle contraction, principally the atrial-ventricular node. This occurs when the triggering of muscle cells in the atrial ventricular node is stronger or more rapid than those from the sino-atrial node. These competing cardiac rhythms are known as arrhythmias. If the electrical activity leading to the production of an R-wave occurs along an unusual path, an ectopic beat results whose shape in an ECG record may differ significantly from normal.

'Intelligent' ECG monitors are able to classify abnormal ECG complexes such as ventricular premature beats (VPB) by storing in memory during a 'learn phase' a software template for a 'normal' beat for that patient at that time and comparing it with each incoming beat. A set of logical rules enables the monitor to log events such as multifocal beats (at least two different VPB shapes since the last learn phase), ventricular tachycardia (at least three successive VPBs with a VPB rate of at least 100 per minute), atrial fibrillation (at least nine successive R-R intervals differ greatly in length), ventricular fibrillation (three seconds of multiple-wide complexes, no normal beats) and asystole (no QRS complex has been detected for more than 3 seconds). The monitor labels and notes the time of occurrence of arrhythmic events and can produce a trend display of these, for example over a period of two hours.

Other types of diagnostic information which can be gained from an electrocardiogram are blockages to the paths of conduction, giving rise to an unusual sequence of events in the P, Q, R, S, T cycle. For example, a left bundle branch block would give rise to an unusual QRS complex, as it is this part of the ECG which corresponds with ventricular contraction. Both the atria and the ventricles can fibrillate: that is to say, they beat in an ineffective uncoordinated fashion. Ventricular fibrillation is life-threatening because of the resulting loss of pumping action and unless corrected promptly (usually by means of an electrical defibrillator) leads to irreversible brain damage or death.

Caution is required in the interpretation of ECGs since the physique of the patient can affect the ECG waveform. In short, plump patients the heart can be pushed up and out by the stomach. In tall, thin, patients, the heart can be positioned more vertically than normal. In both cases, the pathway of conduction can yield apparently abnormal ECG traces.

The electromyogram (EMG) represents the electrical activity of muscle cells in voluntary striated muscle. When a nervous signal activates a muscle, the chain of synchronized action potentials generated along muscle fibres causing them to contract can be picked up by means of surface electrodes placed over the muscle, or by needle electrodes place in the body of the muscle. Diagnostic information obtainable from an EMG includes dysfunction of muscle excitation such as fasciculation and fibrillation.

Fasciculation is a disorder in which an abnormal impulse occurs in a motor nerve fibre causing a contraction which is confined to a localized area. This can sometimes be observed clinically by the presence of a slight ripple in the skin over the affected muscle. Fasciculation is a clinical finding in patients with poliomyelitis, or it can occur following accidents in which nerve fibres innervating the muscle are severely damaged. The typical EMG record in such patients exhibits weak periodic potentials, although these are of sufficient amplitude that they can be picked up by surface electrodes.

In fibrillation of muscle, it is the individual muscle fibre which is affected, and adjacent muscle fibres do not contract. For this reason, fibrillation consisting of spontaneous impulses in denervated muscle fibres can only be recorded by means of needle electrodes. The frequency of fibrillation can be used to deduce the time course of the injury. For three to five days after onset, the frequency of firing is once every few seconds; after one to four weeks this frequency has increased to 3 to 10 Hz; after a further two weeks the muscle fibres atrophy and this produces a cessation of the fibrillation.

The electroencephalogram (EEG) measures the electrical activity of the brain. A major distinguishing feature separating the study of ECGs from EEGs is the fact that the origin and production of the former is well understood, whereas it is still not clear as to how brain waves originate and are produced. What is known regarding the EEG is deduced from empirical evidence that certain patterns in the EEG tracing are signs of particular cerebral dysfunction. The full diagnostic EEG is recorded from a standard 20-electrode array. The location of each electrode is recognized internationally, allowing repeatability of measurement and transfer of data between centres. For routine EEG recording, seven standard combinations (montages) are used, each of eight channels. The measurements are bipolar: that is, the EEG tracing is a record of the time course of the potential differences existing between pairs of electrodes. The advantage of this technique is that any artifact (e.g. from muscle movements) would produce the same effects on both electrodes and these cancel out having little final effect on the recording.

A classification of EEG rhythms groups these into four main classes called: alpha, beta, theta and delta. Alpha rhythm has frequencies in the band 8 to 13 Hz with an amplitude of 10 to 50 microvolts. It can be observed predominantly over the occipital and parieto-occipital areas of the brain, and is diminished by mental or visual activity. Beta rhythm can be recorded from the entire cortex of the brain and lies in the frequency band 16 to 25 Hz with an amplitude rarely exceeding 30 microvolts. Theta rhythms are not usually encountered in normal alert patients, but when they do occur they have frequencies of 4 to 8 Hz with an amplitude of less than 30 microvolts. They can be recorded primarily in the parietal and temporal areas of the brain. Finally, delta rhythm is often seen during sleep and can most easily be recorded from electrodes located near to the vertex. Typically, their frequency range is 0.5 to 3 Hz but their timing is irregular. Their amplitude is high – in excess of 100 microvolts. The diagnostic significance of delta thythm is that intracranial disorders, such as brain tumours, may generate delta rhythms in patients who are awake. Other diagnostic information can be obtained from an EEG by investigating the extent of the abnormalities seen in the recordings. For example, a flashing light stimulus may induce epilepsy in affected individuals where the expectation is that abnormalities will be generated from diffuse areas of the brain, therefore affecting many EEG channels; in contrast, a localized brain tumour will only affect the signal recorded by electrodes situated in the immediate vicinity of the lesion.

Another use made of a single channel EEG recording is in the operating room, where surgeons and anaesthetists may rely on the recording to provide an indication of the patient's cerebral status. If the blood supply to the brain becomes diminished, the tissue becomes hypoxaemic which may have serious consequences. When the patient is unconscious, it is difficult to observe any clinical manifestation of this condition other than the EEG which indicates an abnormal tracing in sufficient time for corrective action to be taken. Automatic EEG analysers are available for use during major surgery for this purpose.

The single channel EEG is also used for the recording of evoked potentials. This is a technique which exists in many forms, but in all cases the electronic averaging of the EEG signal is a key component. The method relies on the response produced in the EEG signal evoked by the known stimulus. The stimulus always occurs after the same interval of time commencing from the start of each recorded time epoch. As the epochs are summated, the time-locked response grows in amplitude, while the background 'noise', if truly random, cancels out. It was the advent of computer-based averaging techniques which revolutionized this area of electrophysiology. Prior to the availability of computer averaging, clinicians employed graphical-summation methods in which only 10 to 20 superimpositions could be used before the measurement became too complex or too long to complete. Another problem with hand-averaged evoked responses occurred with the delineation of the response from the background 'noise' which sometimes is of a greater amplitude than the signal. Typically, 100 one-second epochs of EEG are averaged and the stimulus (auditory, visual or tactile) is presented after 0.2 seconds in each epoch. Evoked response audiometry has been used to diagnose retrocochlear lesions on the VIIIth cranial nerve; brain-stem evoked responses are used to investigate the depth of anaesthesia and also as one of a number of tests to ascertain brain death.

6.5 The choice of recording electrodes

The reliable recording of diagnostic quality bio-electric signals from patients of all ages and all conditions (perspiring, hairy, restless) is essential to routine patient monitoring in intensive care situations and electrophysiological investigations. Typical bio-electric signals encountered during patient monitoring include: the electrocardiogram (ECG), the electroencephalogram (EEG), transcutaneous blood-gas tensions measured with heated electrodes and thoracic-impedance signals for respiration and cardiac output. More specialist investigations can include electromyograms (EMG), nerve-conduction measurements, the electro-occulogram (EOG) and the electroretinogram (ERG).

In some instances the amplitude of the bio-electric signals will be less than 100 microvolts and hence it is important that artifact signals arising from the movement of electrodes, body motion or the pick-up of electrical mains or electrical noise signals must be minimized. Such sources must not give rise to unwanted signals, or if this proves impossible in practice, the equipment must be capable of removing as much of the artifacts as is necessary to leave a clinically acceptable signal. The electrodes must adhere firmly to the skin, but yet be removable without undue discomfort. These requirements have to be seen against the need to monitor patients for extended periods and that they may be hairy, restless and perspiring – in marked contrast to volunteer subjects in a laboratory.

It is important that the site for each electrode is chosen carefully and wherever possible should conform to accepted conventions. A good quality, stable, low noise electrode should be employed, careful preparation of the skin made at the selected site, a non-irritant conducting electrode gel used and the electrode firmly affixed to the skin by means of a non-irritant adhesive. The electrodes should be inspected at regular intervals, particularly in the case of extended periods of patient monitoring, to mitigate against irritation or infection occurring beneath the electrodes and to check that electrodes have not become loosely attached to the skin or disconnected from the input cable of the recording amplifier.

6.6 Requirements for recording electrodes

For the recording of EMG signals from the body of a muscle, fine wire electrodes are employed. The wire is passed through the lumen of a small hypodermic needle and the varnish insulation burned off from the tip using a cigarette lighter. The end of the wire is then bent back over the bevel of the needle to form a hook. The needle is passed through the skin into the muscle and the needle pulled back leaving the wire hooked into the muscle. This technique is useful when recording the EMG of the urethral or anal sphincters. Circular silver/silver chloride surface electrodes are used in rehabilitation studies of leg and arm muscles.

For 12-lead diagnostic ECGs in a cardiology clinic electrode gel is used under metal plate electrodes held in place by rubber straps on the wrist and ankles, plus a set of metal cup suction electrodes placed at standardized locations on the chest wall. After suitable cleaning, these ECG electrodes are reusable. When it is necessary to record a full 12-lead diagnostic ECG from a patient in intensive care, small, square, self-adhesive electrodes suitable for mounting on the chest are available. A metal tag forms one edge of the electrode and this can be connected by means of a spring clip to one lead of the ECG channel's patient cable.

For a good quality diagnostic ECG a bandwidth of 0.05 Hz to 100 Hz is required. The patient is kept as nearly at rest as possible and care is taken in the application of the electrodes. By this means small components of the ECG waveform are faithfully recorded.

For patient-monitoring purposes, as during surgery with diathermy in use or with a restless patient, it may be sufficient to observe only gross changes in the ECG and heart rate. The recording bandwidth can be reduced, e.g. 0.1 to 40 Hz and self-adhesive disposable electrodes employed. A well-known range of disposable electrodes is the Red Dot series by the 3M Company, Figure 6.5. These are based upon the use of a silver/silver chloride-sensing element and are used in conjunction with a solid conducting electrode gel. The Red Dot resting ECG electrode can be held in place with micropore adhesive tape. Its synthetic, polymeric acrylate adhesive provides a secure long-term adhesion and the 100% rayon backing is porous and has a high moisture-vapour transmission rate. 3M quote a skin-electrode contact impedance measured at 10 Hz with the very low mean value of 209 ohms and a mean d.c. offset voltage generated by the electrode on the skin of 0.46 millivolts. To this standing voltage must be added the combined effects of offset instability and internal electrical noise which are given a mean value of zero microvolts by 3M. The EEG is often monitored as one or two channels in order to check that incipient brain damage does not occur during major surgical procedures or that a brain seizure is not threatened. Small disc-shaped chlorided silver electrodes are stuck to prepared sites on the scalp with an adhesive such as collodion.

6.7 The common mode rejection ratio of the recording amplifier

The bioelectric signals detected at the recording electrodes are fed via low electrical noise, well-insulated cables to the active input terminals of a balanced differential amplifier which has a low noise input stage whose input impedance is high (several megohms). For a Lead 1 ECG anti-phase ECG signals are taken from electrodes placed on the right and left wrists and fed into the two active inputs of the ECG amplifier with the right leg electrode acting as the signal earth (indifferent electrode).

The differential amplifier acts to selectively amplify the wanted anti-phase signals while rejecting unwanted in-phase signals such as that due to mains frequency electrical pick-up which bathes the whole of the patient with electromagnetic radiation at 50 Hz (60 Hz in North America).

The common mode rejection ratio (CMRR) of the amplifier is given by $CMRR = (RI/2)/(R1 - R2)$ where RI is the *total* input impedance in ohms between the two active inputs of the amplifier and R1 and R2 are the electrode-skin contact impedances of the two active electrodes in ohms.

If RI = 10 megohms, R1 = 5000 ohms and R2 = 4000 ohms then CMRR = 10 000 so that the wanted signals are amplified 10 000 times more than the unwanted signals. In decibel notation the CMRR = 20 log 10 (10 000) = 20 × 4 = 80 dB. In order to achieve a high value of the CMRR the amplifier must have a high input impedance but also the skin-contact impedances of the recording electrodes must individually be as small as possible and as nearly equal as possible. Thus good skin preparation, the use of conducting electrode gel and firm contact between skin and electrode are important.

6.8 Electrode contact potentials

The voltage picked up from each recording electrode consists of the wanted bio-electric signal usually with unwanted mains-frequency signals and superimposed upon a contact potential consisting of a steady voltage (d.c. offset potential) which may exhibit slow variations (perhaps arising from sweating or temperature changes) and random noise signals. The wanted signal may be periodic in nature, as in the case of the ECG or arterial blood-pressure waveform which follow the cardiac cycle, in which case signal-averaging techniques may be employed to enhance the regular wanted signal against the random background.

The amplitude of the wanted signal may be up to 1000 times smaller than the contact potential which because it is a steady (d.c.) level will not be recorded by an amplifier whose bandwidth does not extend down to 0 Hz. On some situations, such as recording electromyograms from smooth muscle, it may be necessary to record using a bandwidth down to d.c. (0 Hz), but usually a bandwidth extending down to 0.05 Hz is used to eliminate slow drifts in the baseline of the recording. Recording electrodes are carefully designed to produce small, stable and predictable offset potentials which will not overload the input stage of the recording amplifier or generate noise 'spikes' which could be recorded.

6.9 Reversible electrodes

The combination of a metal electrode and an electrolyte (tissue fluid) forms a half-cell which generates a d.c. potential whose magnitude depends on both the nature of the metal and the electrolyte. A combination of electrode and electrolyte for which the offset voltage between a pair of recording electrodes is zero when no current is drawn (because each has acquired the same potential) is known as a reversible cell. Silver chloride is most suitable as a stable recording material for bioelectric signals. The approximation to reversibility is confirmed by the fact that potential differences of only a fraction of a millivolt can exist between pairs of carefully prepared silver/silver chloride electrodes. A good example of a modern silver/silver chloride ECG monitoring electrode occurs with the Red Dot neonatal-monitoring electrode by 3M Health Care, Figure 6.5. Each disc

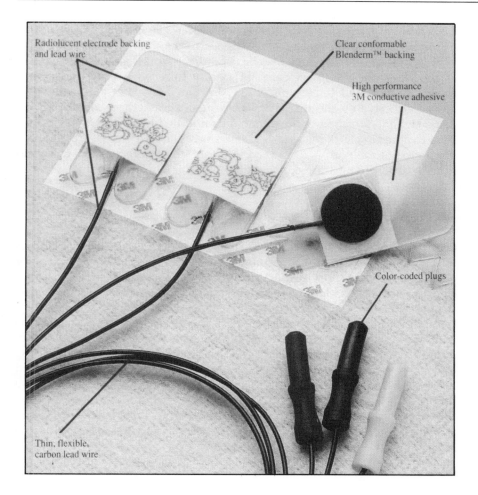

Radiolucent electrode backing
and lead wire

Clear conformable
Blenderm™ backing

High performance
3M conductive adhesive

Color-coded plugs

Thin, flexible,
carbon lead wire

Figure 6.5 Red Dot Neonatal ECG Monitoring Electrode. (Courtesy 3M Health Care.)

electrode is provided with a pre-attached thin, flexible, carbon-lead wire, a long-lasting conductive adhesive, an electrode backing which is opaque to X-rays and a wider transparent backing to allow for a continuous inspection of the skin.

6.10 Skin preparation

A good preparation of the skin which is to underlie the recording electrode is important particularly in adults where the skin may possess quite a tough outer horny layer. A hair-free site should be chosen if possible, or hair removed from the site. It may be possible to locate the electrode in a position with little underlying muscle in order to minimize myoelectric signals from the muscle during exercise. The outer horny layer of skin should be abraded with pumice and an ether-methylated spirit mixture used to degrease the skin. A non-irritant (low chloride) conducting electrode gel is rubbed into the prepared area of skin and the electrode firmly bedded into the gel and then affixed to the skin.

Sticky (Sellotape) tape can also be used to strip off the outer horny layer of the skin. The manufacturers 3M Health Care have produced a tape especially designed for the purpose – 3M One Step Skin Prep. This tape has an adhesive on the rear surface. A one-inch length is taken from the dispenser and attached to the attendant's middle finger. The finger is then used to abrade selected electrode sites using a moderate pressure and only one swipe of the pad. It is claimed that this simple preparation will yield skin-electrode contact impedances of approximately 10 000 ohms.

6.11 Adhesion of electrodes to the skin

Collodion is used as an adhesive to attach small chlorided silver electrodes to the patient's scalp to form a montage of electrodes. ECG electrodes for patient-monitoring purposes are affixed to the chest and can consist of a chlorided silver disc mounted inside a small plastic cup provided with a flange. The disc is connected with a male press-stud which protrudes through the rear of the cup to mate with the female portion located at the end of the connecting cable. The cup is filled with contact gel and acts to minimize motion between the gel and the skin. Pre-gelled disposable ECG electrodes using a solid gel are available, such as the Red Dot Clear Backed Electrodes from 3M Health Care, Figure 6.6. These are designed to have a low profile in order to minimize tugging by clothing or drapes and are provided with a strong adhesive and a non-porous flexible backing which is impervious to fluids which can penetrate and interfere with the adhesion to the skin.

Figure 6.6 Red Dot ECG Monitoring Electrode. (Courtesy 3M Health Care.)

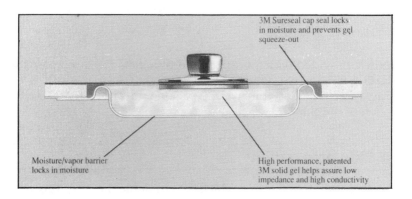

The elements of patient-monitoring systems

7

7.1 Introduction

The use of sensors, electrodes and their associated signal-processing and display techniques has become widespread in high dependency patient areas of hospitals for the routine monitoring of vital signs and other variables as an aid to managing patients who are often in a markedly unstable condition. The ranges within which a particular variable might be considered 'normal' and the format of the display may often be determined by the medical staff. The equipment may be serviced by hospital clinical engineers or by the supplier's service staff. However, nursing staff are likely to be particularly involved in observing the data produced and ensuring that it remains valid and is not corrupted by events such as blood clotting in a cannula. This is particularly true out of normal daylight working hours.

Computers are steadily increasing in power while shrinking in size. At the same time there have been distinct advances made in digital-display technology enabling the user to have access to a variety of text, numerical data and graphic displays, often in colour. The computing power available makes it feasible to calculate real-time statistics from the incoming data, to apply digital filtering to raw data and to generate three-dimensional displays where this would assist the observer in the interpretation of the patient's condition. Digital data links are now well-established and can be used to link bedside patient monitors to a central nursing station. The raw signals from recording electrodes and transducers are known as analogue signals and they vary continuously with time. By sampling the analogue signal and storing its value at preset intervals, the analogue signal is converted into digital form i.e. a series of discrete values which can be stored and processed in a computer.

However sophisticated the processing, the old adage 'garbage in, garbage out' still applies and it is vital to ensure that the original signals are of good quality. The site in or on the patient's body from which the original signal is obtained determines the electrical safety requirements for that particular signal channel. For example, when signals have to be recorded directly from the heart, the most stringent electrical safety precautions must be observed, whereas these can be relaxed within specified limits when recording from the surface of the body. These are discussed in detail in Chapter 15.

7.2 Electrodes and transducers

The variables of interest in patient monitoring are either of an electrical nature, such as the electrocardiogram (ECG), in which case they are obtained via electrodes located on the patient, or they exist as physical occurrences e.g. the arterial blood pressure and need transforming into a corresponding electrical signal which can be fed into an appropriate pre-amplifier. A transducer is a device which transduces (transforms) the physiological variable into the corresponding electrial signal; for example, the application of an arterial blood pressure is caused to move a diaphragm whose motion is converted into an electrical signal whose variation with time corresponds with that of the blood pressure.

Electrodes are constructed from suitable materials and made in such a form that they enable a stable signal to be picked up; they are compatible with the patient and can be used for extended periods if necessary. A wide range of transducers is available, including types for blood-pressure recording, body-temperature measurement, respiratory gas flow and composition and blood-gas tensions and oxygen saturation.

Transducers will have to be chosen with the particular clinical circumstances in mind, e.g. a paediatric blood-pressure cuff for use with non-invasive blood-pressure measurements on children, or a large pneumotachograph head for use with patients during exercise-tolerance tests in contrast to a smaller head suitable for gas-flow studies conducted on anaesthetized patients. Transducers tend to be expensive and must be handled and stored with consideration if their function and calibration is to be maintained. They are also likely to be in contact with patient fluids and must be disinfected according to the manufacturer's instructions before use with the next patient. Autoclaving to achieve sterility can permanently damage many types of transducer.

7.3 Pre-amplifiers

In a conventional patient-monitoring system there is a set of pre-amplifiers, each designed to handle a particular patient variable. An ECG amplifier will have a bandwidth which extends from 0.05 Hz to some 100 Hz. It does not go down to d.c. in order to avoid very low frequency artifacts such as those generated by patient movement or sweating. The pre-amplifier may also contain filters for modifying the waveform of the recorded signal. As an example, for the purposes of only monitoring the general shape of the ECG a filter can usually be switched in to limit the upper 3 dB cut-off frequency to 40 Hz and thus reduce the effect of higher frequencies appearing in the form of noise on the ECG. The pre-amplifiers will provide a standard 1 millivolt amplitude calibration signal and a gain control to adjust the displayed ECG to a standard sensitivity such as 1 mV per cm. More elaborate filtering may be performed subsequently by passing the recorded signal through digital (software) filters.

An interesting example of filtering occurs in the recording of the electro-gastrogram (EGG) – the gastric myoelectric activity of the stomach recorded from abdominal surface electrodes with pressure activities of the distal stomach and upper small bowel recorded by means of an intralu-minal pressure probe (Chen, J., McCallum, R. W. and Richards, R. (1993)) 'Frequency components of the electrogastrogram and their correlations with gastrointestinal contractions in humans', *Medical and Biological Engineering and Computing*, **31**, 60–6. The recording frequency range for the stomach pressure variations was set at 0-0.3 Hz and the low and high cut-off frequencies for the electrogastrogram were set at 0.02 Hz and 0.3 Hz respectively. To observe more clearly superimposed low and high frequency components present in the EGG, some of the recordings were further filtered by means of digital filters. A digital low-pass filter was used to filter out any activities with frequencies higher than 1.2 cycles per minute and a high-pass filter with a cut-off frequency of 6 cycles per minute was used to filter out any activities with frequencies of lower than 6 cycles per minute and to bring out any superimposed high frequency component of about 12 cycles per minute.

The pre-amplifier also acts as an 'impedance transformer' to provide a high input impedance to interface with the recording electrodes and to provide an output at a lower impedance suitable for driving a recorder. A pressure transducer pre-amplifier might provide an amplitude stabilized audio-frequency signal capable of energizing inductive or resistive pressure transducers. It will have a gain control to enable the pressure calibration to be adjusted against a known pressure or an electronic calibration signal.

Manufacturers of patient-monitor systems provide a full range of pre-amplifiers which can be assembled to cater for the particular clinical circumstances. Each pre-amplifier provides a standard level of output signal which can be fed into identical main amplifiers which will drive a display, perhaps an ink jet recorder. An isolator stage may be interposed between the pre- and main amplifier to provide electrical isolation in order to protect the patient from any risk of a micro-shock. Instead of being fed into a main amplifier as in an analogue system, the conditioned signals can be fed into an analogue-to-digital converter where the amplitude of the analogue signal is sampled at a pre-determined rate. The resulting series of digital values of the amplitude, each taken at a known time, is passed to a computer for processing, storage and display.

The Nyquist sampling theorem requires that the sampling rate should be at least twice the upper bandwidth limit frequency in order that the resulting series of digital values faithfully represents the original analogue signal. For example, a diagnostic ECG signal bandwidth of 0.05 Hz to 100 Hz would require an analogue-to-digital conversion rate of at least 200 per second. In practice 300 per second might be used. The sampling rate may be under the control of a personal computer and it is important to be certain that an adequate sampling rate has been set into the software and that adequate data storage has been provided appropriate to the sampling rate and the period of sampling.

7.4 Amplifier considerations

The combination of pre-amplifier and main amplifier used to detect and display bioelectric signals such as the ECG and EEG is quite sophisticated in design. This must conform with international standards for stray electrical leakage currents to and from the patient. There must be a high value of common mode rejection ratio in order to discriminate against unwanted signals with particular reference to mains-frequency interference. The input impedance must be high, typically at least 2.5 megohms, in order to minimize distortion of the bio-electric signal arising from the electrodes making a relatively poor contact with the patient. The bandwidth of the amplifier must be adequate for the purpose, i.e. it should be able to handle the range of frequencies required to produce the desired amount of detail in the waveform of the bio-electric signal, typically 0.5 to 25 Hz for ECG monitoring and 0.05 to 100 Hz for a diagnostic ECG recording. The linearity and dynamic range of the amplifier's response must be able to cope with the full range of amplitudes of the signal's components without distoring the waveform due to overloading. An ECG amplifier should be able to display cardiac-pacemaker pulses whose amplitude may be several hundred times greater than that of the ECG. In this case an automatic gain control is required to limit the gain of the amplifier so that pacemaker signals will not overload a mechanical device such as a pen recorder and cause damage.

The amplifiers discussed so far are designed to faithfully reproduce the ECG waveform. Sometimes a tuned amplifier designed only to respond to a limited range of frequencies is required, for example, to respond to the QRS complex of the ECG and to count the complexes in order to determine the heart rate. In order to trigger a cardiac pacemaker, an amplifier is required which will detect P and R-waves and which passes frequencies of 20 to 40 Hz but will exclude T-waves (0.7 to 2 Hz) and EMG activity (70 to 500 Hz).

7.5 Displays

Patient-monitor systems now provide comprehensive alphanumeric (text) and graphics on a cathode ray tube, plasma screen or liquid-crystal display, Figure 7.1. The text portion of the display will provide the patient's identification details, time and date and numerical values such as heart rate, blood pressure(s), respiration rate and body temperature and an indication of threshold limits for alarms. The graphical portion will provide a number of possibilities, such as a representation of ECG and arterial blood-pressure tracings and trend plots showing the changes over time of selected patient variables such as heart rate and blood pressure.

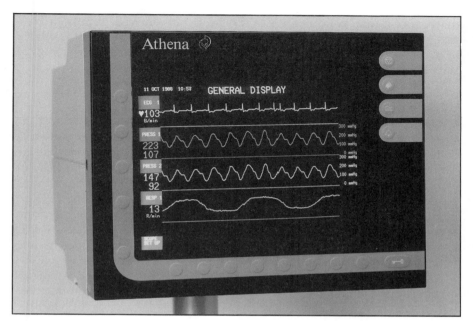

Figure 7.1 Typical patient monitor display of the ECG, two Arterial Blood Pressures and Respiration. (Courtesy S & W Vickers Ltd.)

The primary analogue signals from the pre-amplifiers will have been digitized (converted to a corresponding series of sampled values at rates of typically 300 per second for the ECG and 100 per second for arterial blood pressure). A set of discrete values is stored in the patient-monitor's computer memory and recalled as required for display on the screen in the form of a set of 'frozen' traces. This provision of a stationary tracing facilitates the diagnosis of events such as a cardiac arrhythmia. The contents of the screen display can be dumped on to a printer-plotter to provide a hard copy and also on to a magnetic disc for storage.

7.6 Alarms

In principle it is desirable that a patient-monitor system can alert staff when the values of selected variables move outside predetermined settings. Both audible and visual alarms can usually be activated. If a remote alarm facility is available, for example at a central nursing station, it is important that the alarm can only be cancelled by staff returning to the main monitor by the bedside in order that they can then check on the patient's condition and ascertain the cause of the alarm. This is part of a wider philosophy in which nurses always refer back to the patient and do not trust only in information displayed on monitor screens.

False alarms rapidly reduce staff confidence in the system and can upset patients. Restless or perspiring patients often cause ECG electrodes to become loose on the skin and generate movement artifact signals which give rise to an apparent tachycardia. Scrupulous care in the siting and preparation of electrodes is vital. False heart rate alarms can be substantially reduced by requiring that a tachycardia alarm is set only by the meeting of a dual condition e.g. a fast heart rate derived from both ECG and blood pressure signals. It may also be desirable that a patient is unable to observe a visual alarm since this may trigger an unstable physiological state due to insecurity of the patient.

7.7 Variables monitored

The variables most commonly monitored are the ECG, blood pressure, body temperature and oxygen saturation. In obstetric situations uterine contractions and maternal and foetal heart rates will be monitored. In cardiac surgery the ECG, a number of blood pressures, body temperatures at several sites and in the extracorporeal circulation and often the EEG (to monitor cerebral function) are monitored. For patients suffering from respiratory insufficiency in addition to the ECG and blood pressure it is usual to monitor variables such as respiratory rate, tidal and minute volume and oxygen saturation.

As a general rule, it pays to invest in good quality, user-friendly patient-monitoring systems from a well-established and approved manufacturer with a proven service capability. The system must be capable of handling all the commonly encountered physiological variables and be capable of expansion to take on new variables when these are introduced.

7.8 Trend plots

Trend-plot facilities are often provided with patient-monitoring systems and can be particularly useful in showing the build-up of cardiac arrhythmias or changes in blood pressure over periods of time such as the previous 24 hours. Automatic adaptation of the scale ranges provides a clear display if there is a wide range of values for a particular variable. The nature and time of specific events can be annotated on the display, together with details of interventions such as medication. Figure 7.2 illustrates a typical trend-function display incorporating trends in arterial oxygen percentage saturation, electrocardiogram and two blood pressures.

7.9 Portable patient monitors for use with patient-transport systems

Circumstances regularly arise in which it is important to be able to continue the monitoring of a patient who is being moved from one location to another, e.g. from the scene of an accident to a hospital by ambulance or helicopter or from the operating theatre to the intensive care unit.

Monitors such as the PROPAQ 106, Figure 7.3, have been specially developed which are light in weight (less than 10 lb including pulse oximetry), have a low power consumption electroluminescent display for waveforms and alphanumeric data and can operate from a self-contained rechargeable battery pack for up to ten hours. The carrying handle is

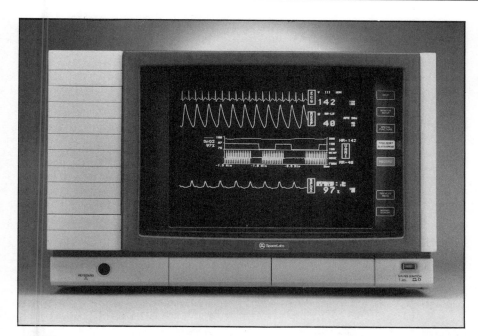

Figure 7.2 A patient-monitor display showing physiological waveforms (ECG, Respiration and Oxygen Saturation) together with a trend display of these three variables. (Courtesy Spacelabs Medical Inc.)

curved to allow the monitor to be hung from a trolley or bed rail. A compressor is provided for use with non-invasive blood-pressure measurements or two pressure transducers can be plugged in as can a pulse oximeter pick-up. The ECG is detected from disposable self-adhesive electrodes and a small strip-chart recorder provides hard copy. Sufficient numerical data can be stored in memory to provide five-hour trend plots.

An alternative approach allows a multiparameter module from a bedside-patient monitor to be removed and plugged into a portable battery-pack housing to form a portable monitor which can move with the patient on a trolley, so preserving continuity of monitoring techniques while the patient is on the move within the hospital.

7.10 The use of a central station

Individual patient monitors are normally provided with a digital signal output port which conforms to an international format such as RS 232 and which can feed its signals into a local area network (LAN) which often runs on a protocol such as Ethernet, see Section 2.6.4 of Chapter 2. The network can feed information from a number of individual monitors to a central display console which is often located at the unit's nursing station. If analogue signals are also available as outputs, these are normalized to a one-volt amplitude corresponding with the full scale for that channel. The analogue signals are sent to a central analogue display or tape recorder via multi-way cable. A typical example occurs with a four-or six-bed coronary care unit.

It is desirable that patients should not continuously observe their own monitor's display since the presence of ectopic beats on the ECG waveform may give rise to concern to the patient and induce further runs of ectopics. Central

Figure 7.3 PROPAQ 106
portable patient monitor.
(Courtesy Protocol Systems Inc.)

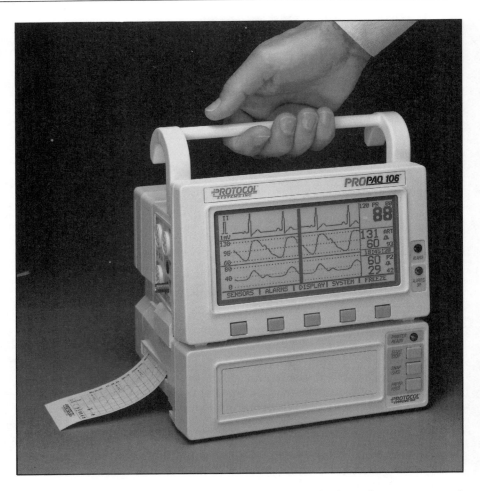

stations are usually provided with a strip recorder which can be programmed
to record from selected monitors on request or to a pre-set schedule.

7.11 Patient data-management systems

The critically ill patient requires more clinical information for a successful
outcome than does a conventional hospital patient. The complexity of the
information is high as it is necessary to integrate data from various sources
and of numerous types. As well as physiological variables from the
patient, data-management systems for intensive care purposes must record
items from the clinical and nursing record, therapy decisions and plans,
laboratory data, administrative data and reports from other relevant
departments. Technology has also increased to such an extent that data
processing and interpretation must take place in real time in order to cope
with the rapid production of information from on-line measurements. In
an intensive care unit it is typical to collect, process, store and display up
to 1000 items of data per patient per day. This is very time consuming for

nurses and demands a high attention span for prolonged periods. Work studies have revealed that up to one-third of nursing time in an ICU can be spent on the keeping of records and charting of patients. It is becoming possible to capture electronically most of the patient data set, and where this approach is used, a marked evolution of patient-management strategies has occurred due to the increase in the available information. This in turn leads to improved patient management and outcomes.

Developments in patient-management protocols have occurred alongside developments in other fields which affect patient outcome, notably: the development of new surgical procedures; the development of new therapies; the use of novel instrumentation systems to monitor the therapy and the increase in general measurement technology which includes the use of microprocessor or computer-based procedures. It is possible to trace the evolution of patient data-management systems using five phases to describe their continuous development. Phase one is the simple bedside monitor whose function is just to monitor vital signs. Limit alarms may be provided to indicate when the monitored signal strays outside preset acceptable limits. In Phase two is an increase in instrument technology which has led to more sophisticated bedside monitors. These have more channels and allow comparison of the time-dependent behaviour of several physiological variables from which derived variables can be calculated, for example, an estimate of cardiac work from the mean arterial blood pressure and the cardiac output. It has also become possible to review historical trends in variables to provide an indication of the response of the patient to therapy. The number of variables which could be measured has gradually increased, leading to a requirement for more sophisticated and complex technology. An integrated approach to the management of patient data was sought: the bedside monitor became one element of a wider system for computer-based data management. Other elements include the automatic lung ventilator, blood-gas analyser and infusion pumps.

Thus the third phase comprises a patient data-management system for each ICU bed. Each system is capable of monitoring, trending, storing and displaying patient data with automatic reporting arrangements and simple calculations being available in the more advanced versions. Whereas in phase three the patient data management system was unique to each bed, in phase four further integration and communication between computers became possible. Networks of computers allow data processing at the bedside and storage of data at some central facility. Not only is most of the data collected automatically, freeing the nurses from much clerical work, but clinicians can now review all the patients in the ward from one site. Most commercial data-management systems are now in this stage of development. However, a fifth phase can be identified which requires a methodological rather than a technological change. The data-processing function of earlier systems has led, in some cases, to systems which are able to interpret data. Technically, the outcome of this further transformation results in patient information-management systems.

These aim to be helpful both to the clinical user and in the provision of increased care for the patient; to be sufficiently flexible for the effect of upgrades to medical equipment to insignificantly affect the operation of the overall system; to reduce the amount of paper produced to the extent that a paperless intensive care unit becomes possible; and to assist in the process of clinical audit.

Advantages accruing from the use of a patient data-management system include the automated recording of data and automated data management from a range of different monitoring and therapy devices. However, many intensive care units currently rely on older models of equipment which do not possess a digital communication port. This disadvantage will gradually reduce as equipment is replaced with compatible modern versions. An example of a commercial patient data-management system is the CareVue 9000 system from Hewlett Packard. This comprises a network of 32 computers in a Star topology (Chapter 2). There is a 'clinical workstation' (computer, VDU and keyboard) located at each bedside and this, together with the patient monitor, is linked via a serial data network to CD-WORM (Write Only Read Many times) drives where the data are recorded. Off-line data, such as observations made by nurses, are entered from the bedside keyboards. Data may be validated (that is, accepted by the user) at intervals which have a minimum resolution of one minute, although in practice this is likely to be one hour. The amount of data stored is greatly reduced, since only validated data are written to the CD-WORM drive.

Figure 7.4(a) illustrates a scheme based on the latest technology – which can be seen in use in Figure 7.4(b). The patient's chart is replaced by a computer equivalent database. The clinician or nurse can query the database (dotted lines represent a query) only via the so-called 'human-computer interface'. The usual interface for data input is the keyboard, but other methods for manual data entry are under investigation. Electronic pointing devices, such as the mouse or trackerball, are becoming popular in clinical versions of patient data-management systems. Data-output techniques involve VDUs or printers. Manufacturers are aware of the attraction of colour displays.

The more advanced patient data-management systems provide 'decision support'. This is a computer-based system which can mimic the reasoning strategies of experienced intensivists. Decision support encompasses the use of knowledge regarding data management, alarm states, therapy critique and the use of intelligent interfaces to other medical equipment.

There are various forms of knowledge models used in the implementation of decision-support systems including patient-specific models, mathematical models and expert systems. A patient-specific model attempts to cover the relevant pathophysiological processes independently for each patient. In order for a particular type of implementation to be successful, the physiological dysfunction should be well-defined and lead to a set of unambiguous treatment regimes. Mathematical modelling can be used to describe, explain, predict or control pathophysiological processes based on models constructed from differential equations. In some cases, these equations are easy to comprehend, for example, at a gross level: Fluid Balance = Fluid In - Fluid Out.

'Fluid In' can be determined by those responsible for the management of the patient, but 'Fluid Out' is more complicated, since as well as measuring

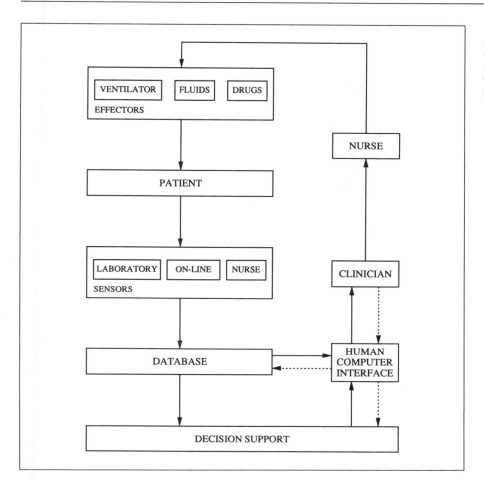

Figure 7.4 The integration of decision support into patient data-management systems: **(a)** flowchart; **(b)** shown in use on the Hewlett Packard Care ZUE 9000 Clinical Information System. (By courtesy of Hewlett Packard Ltd.)

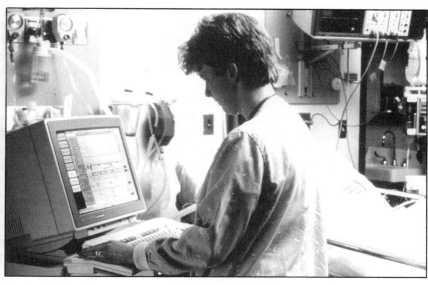

urine and faeces, mathematical terms have to be defined for insensible losses such those due to transpiration (sweating). It is therefore easy to obtain a very complicated mathematical expression for a fairly simple physiological concept. To simplify the mathematical model of a physiological process, aggregation, abstraction or idealization of concepts are often required. For example, it may be mathematically expedient to ignore fluid losses other than those in urine and faeces, knowing that the value obtained for 'Fluid Out' is going to be an underestimate, but still sufficiently accurate for the purposes of the model.

Expert systems use more direct representations of knowledge in the form of IF ... THEN production rules, for example:

IF   tidal volume is less than the pre-set minimum
OR   partial pressure of end-tidal carbon dioxide is greater than 55 mm Hg (7.31 kPa)
THEN   the patient is insufficiently ventilated

This knowledge rule gives two conditions from which it can be concluded that the patient is insufficiently ventilated. A further rule in the knowledge base would then be invoked to indicate which course of action should be taken. This particular example is discussed in more detail in Chapter 8. For such systems to work at a truly expert level, the knowledge which is entered must be provided by experienced clinicians. A set of techniques for eliciting the knowledge has evolved, as it was found that some expert knowledge is implicit and difficult to divulge to others.

As well as modelling expert-level knowledge, expert systems have to mimic how to handle the knowledge stored in their 'electronic brain'. Most reasoning strategies follow the 'test and hypothesize' cycle: that is, they hypothesize about a particular situation with elements from their knowledge base. If this knowledge helps in solving the problem, then a conclusion can be drawn; if it does not help, then an alternative hypothesis is tested using different elements in the knowledge base. This approach may seem very mechanistic, but it must be remembered that the computer processing can be very fast. In most applications of expert systems, when no more conclusions can be drawn, additional data are requested from the user.

Expert systems have been implemented for diagnosis and therapy planning, as well as for the diagnosis of faults in the medical technology surrounding the patient. A limitation of this approach lies in its acceptance by the medical profession. There are good reasons why, although many experts' systems have been implemented, only a few are in actual daily clinical use. In most cases, the knowledge encapsulated by the expert system fails to work consistently at a sufficiently high level for clinical dependence; in some cases the interface between the clinical user and the expert system lacks sophistication; in other cases a lack of trust in the technology is cited as a reason for their non-acceptance. It can only be a matter of time before all these constraints can be relaxed, ensuring a transition to phase five and the evolution of patient information-management systems.

Automatic lung ventilators and humidifiers

8

8.1 The ventilator as a life-support system

The role of an automatic lung ventilator is that of a reliable machine providing an adequate tidal flow of air or other gas/anaesthetic vapour mixture to the patient's lungs at the necessary respiratory rate when the patient is unable to perform this function for himself or herself.

Depending on the degree of respiratory insufficiency, if augmentation of the natural respiration is not undertaken, hypoxia or anoxia can result with serious consequences. Hence the reliability of the functioning of an automatic lung ventilator is vital as is the continuity of its power source, be it the electrical mains, battery, gas pipeline or gas cylinder. Should the ventilator lose its power supply completely it must be possible either to operate the ventilator by hand until the power is restored or to manually ventilate the patient using a spring-loaded rubber bag in conjunction with a facemask and breathing valve. Mainline ventilators are normally fitted with a built-in rechargeable battery to power the ventilator when the normal supply is disconnected.

Similarly, the connection of the ventilator to the patient is vital. Patients are often restless and disoriented, leading to the disconnection of the ventilator tubing which connects to a tracheostomy tube or facemask or they may try to pull the facemask away from their face. Adequate observation of ventilated patients supplemented by ventilator alarms is important.

The use of suitable filters should prevent the patient from being ventilated with contaminated air and the spread of infection from the patient's expired gases. Care will be needed to check that the filters have not become clogged with deposited water from the expirate. Those circuits through which the patient's expired gases pass should be easily detachable and capable of being autoclaved or disinfected as instructed in the user's operating manual.

Automatic lung ventilators operate on the principle of intermittent positive pressure ventilation, a positive pressure applied to the entrance of the airway pushing the required tidal volume into the patient's airway and lungs. The amount of gas delivered per 1 cm water of additional pressure applied is known as the patient's compliance. For the intact chest a typical total compliance (chest wall plus rib cage plus lungs) is 50 cc per 1 cm water (0.511 litres per kilopascal). Thus the application of 10 cm water pressure would deliver a tidal volume of 500 cc. A test lung used to evaluate the performance in the laboratory of automatic lung ventilators might have a compliance of 0.2 litres per kilopascal (19.6 cc per 1 cm of water) and an airways resistance of 2 kilopascals per litre per second (20.5 cm of water per litre per second).

8.2 Types of commonly encountered ventilator

Compact ventilators which are often powered from a gas cylinder or pipeline are commonplace in hospitals mounted on anaesthetic machines or by individual beds in intensive care units. Versions using pneumatic logic control circuitry can be sufficiently small to allow mounting of the ventilator in the cabin of an emergency medical service helicopter, power being provided by oxygen cylinders mounted at the rear of the cabin. Larger models of ventilator, usually with a motor-driven gas compressor and electric mains/battery supply, are used in intensive care units for patients requiring longer term ventilation – possibly for several days or more.

The simpler ventilators apply a constant pressure of several centimetres of water to the input to the patient's airway for a preset time in order to deliver the required tidal volume. At the end of the inspiratory period (perhaps two seconds) the entrance to the patient's airway is switched to the room atmosphere allowing the inflation pressure to decrease exponentially to atmospheric pressure. This is so-called passive expiration. The ventilator is then automatically changed over to the inspiratory mode and the ventilatory cycle repeats continuously, Figure 3.1.

This is a 'pressure-generator' type of ventilator. A report (Handelsman, H. (1991) 'Intermittent Positive Pressure Breathing Therapy', Health Technology Assessment Reports No. 1, US Department of Health and Human Services, Office of Health Technology Assessment, Rockville, Maryland MD 20857, USA) describes the use of intermittent positive pressure breathing using pressure-generator type devices to deliver a controlled pressure of a gas to assist in ventilation or expansion of the lungs and also for the delivery of medication in aerosol form. Handelsman makes the point that in studies, intermittent positive pressure breathing has been shown to have unequivocal clinical effectiveness in terms of morbidity, mortality or lung function.

The larger models of ventilator employed a powerful compressor capable of producing perhaps 100 cm of water pressure. This is substantially greater than the back pressure which builds up in the lungs during inflation as a consequence of the elastance of the lungs, rib cage and chest wall. Hence, there is a more or less constant rate of gas flow into the lungs which does not now fall off due to the build-up of back pressure in the lungs and we speak of a 'constant flow' generator. The flow diminishes exponentially with the simpler constant pressure generator because the inflation pressure is then not much higher than the pressure in the lungs.

Young and Sykes (Young, J. D. and Sykes M. K. (1991) 'Artificial ventilation: history, equipment and techniques' in *Assisted Ventilation* (ed.) J. Moxham, London, *British Medical Journal*, 1–13) make the point that flow generators are generally used with adults and pressure generators with children or with adults where the control of peak airway pressure is important. Young and Sykes find that a pressure generator is particularly useful in children where uncuffed endotracheal tubes are used and there is a leak of gas around the endotracheal tube during inspiration. A pressure generator will tend to compensate for the leak by increasing the gas flow into the airway. With a flow generator under these circumstances a proportion of the tidal volume will be lost to the leak.

8.3 Cycling

An automatic lung ventilator, as the name implies, continuously and automatically changes over from the inspiratory to the expiratory mode and vice versa. This changeover (cycling) can be initiated on a pressure, volume or time basis or combinations of these. With pressure cycling, a pressure sensor monitors the airway pressure and trips the ventilator over to the expiratory phase when a preset pressure has been reached. Passive expiration to room atmosphere may then be allowed for a preset time after which the ventilator changes over to inspiration and so on.

Alternatively, a volume-measuring device such as a bellows spirometer or a turbine respirometer can be used to monitor the delivered inspiratory tidal volume. When a preset volume has been attained, the ventilator automatically changes over to expiration. The volume-measuring device should be located on the expiratory side of the tubing connecting to and from the patient. Then, even if leaks have occurred in the connections on the inspiratory side of the circuit, the patient must have received a tidal volume at least equal to that recorded by the monitoring device.

The principle of time cycling is used in the minute volume divider type of ventilator which is much used in conjunction with anaesthetic machines. By means of the flowmeters on the anaesthetic machine an adequate minute volume of gas mixture is established, perhaps three litres of oxygen plus three litres of nitrous oxide per minute. The ventilator might 'chop' this up into 12 breaths per minute each of 500 cc tidal volume, each delivered over an inspiration time of two seconds, followed by an expiration time of three seconds. Such a minute volume divider is colloquially known as a 'flow chopper'.

8.4 Patient triggering

A ventilator normally cycles repetitively from inspiration to expiration. This is straightforward when the patient is apnoeic, as when a muscle-relaxant agent is in use during anaesthesia, but there may be a problem of competing rhythms when the patient's natural pattern of spontaneous respiration clashes with the imposed ventilatory pattern of the ventilator. It is then useful to switch the ventilator into its triggered mode. Here, a pressure sensor detects the small negative pressure produced by the patient in attempting an inspiration. This effect is arranged to change the ventilator over to the inspiratory mode and causes the ventilator to back-up the patient's attempted inspiration with the delivery of a full tidal volume. The triggering facility is valuable in helping to wean a patient off the ventilator back to fully spontaneous respiration, perhaps following the injection of an antagonist to reverse the paralytic action of a muscle-relaxant agent.

Pressure supported ventilation (PSV) is a mode of ventilation in which the patient triggers the ventilator which takes over the work of respiration from the patient who may be feeble by providing pressure support during inspiration. PSV can be combined with synchronized intermittent manda-tory ventilation (SIMV) to provide pressure support during spontaneous breathing, together with volume-controlled breaths at regular intervals.

There is the danger that if a patient's attempts at spontaneous respira-tion fade away he could receive zero ventilation. Hence in the triggered mode the ventilator must always provide a basal level of ventilation in case the patient stops breathing on his or her own. This is known as inter-mittent mandatory ventilation (IMV). There is no synchronization between the spontaneous breaths and those delivered by the ventilator. As a result it can happen that a patient will take a spontaneous breath and then receive a mandatory breath from the ventilator before he has exhaled completely. The result is a large tidal volume leading to a high peak airway pressure. This phenomenon is called 'stacking'. It can be avoided by using a synchronized mode in which when a mandatory breath was due the ventilator waits until the patient inspires and then delivers the mandatory breath so that the two coincide.

8.5 Expiratory modes

When the patient is allowed to expire passively through the ventilator to the room the expiratory condition is known as zero end-expiratory pressure (ZEEP), where the room atmospheric pressure is taken as zero, Figure 8.1.

By placing the end of the expiratory hose under water or by means of a spring-loaded valve, the end-expiratory pressure can be maintained at some preset pressure of a few cm of water above atmospheric in order to prevent the lungs from collapsing. This technique is known as positive end-expiratory pressure (PEEP), Figure 8.2.

When suction is applied during expiration to draw gas out of the lungs, perhaps via a narrow endotracheal tube as in children, the technique is known as negative end-expiratory pressure (NEEP), Figure 8.3.

Shapiro, S. H., Ernst, P., Gray-Donald, K., Martin, J. G., Wood-

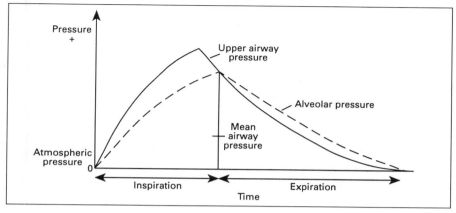

Figure 8.1 Upper airway pressure variations with time during one cycle of a pressure generator type of ventilator.

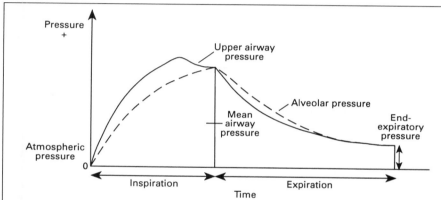

Figure 8.2 Upper airway pressure variations with time during a ventilatory cycle when a positive end-expiratory pressure is used.

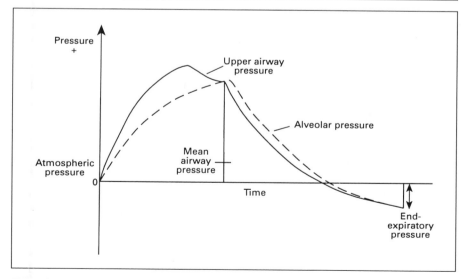

Figure 8.3 Upper airway pressure variations with time during a ventilatory cycle when the ventilator develops a negative pressure phase during expiration.

Dauphinee, S., Beaupre, A., Spitzer, W. O. and Macklem, P. T. (1992) 'Effect of negative pressure ventilation in severe chronic obstructive pulmonary disease', *The Lancet*, **340**, 1425–9 and an editorial in the same issue (p. 1440) point out that NEEP was not efficacious with patients suffering from that particular condition.

On the more sophisticated models of ventilator it is readily possible to select any one of these modes as required.

8.6 End-inspiratory pause

Facilities are often provided to hold the ventilator in the inspiratory mode for a preset period following the cessation of inspiration. This pause allows the pressure in the lungs to equilibrate with the airway pressure so that the airway-pressure gauge-reading now corresponds with the pressure in the lungs, Figure 8.4.

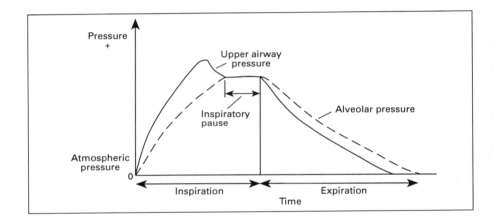

Figure 8.4 The use of an inspiratory pause with a ventilator to allow the upper airway and alveolar pressures to equilibrate.

8.7 The use of artificial sighs

A facility is often provided to generate an extra large tidal volume at intervals of a preset number of breaths. Sighs occur in spontaneous respiration and are thought to be physiologically necessary.

8.8 The use of room air filters and bacterial filters

It is desirable for the air taken in by a ventilator to be passed through a particulate filter to prevent dust and grit particles from entering the mechanism of the ventilator and the patient's airways and lungs. A pleated type of bacterial filter should be fitted to the expired gas port of the ventilator to prevent cross-infection arising from the passage of bacteria from the patient's expired gases contaminating the room atmosphere. The filter may be electrically heated from a low voltage supply to prevent the condensation of expired water vapour. It is important that the supplier's instructions be followed in regard to the servicing of ventilator filters.

8.9 Power sources for ventilators

Ventilators of the portable variety may be powered from air or oxygen cylinders but those used during anaesthesia, in intensive care units or in wards, are normally powered from hospital pipelines. In the case of cylinders it is important to ensure that replacements are readily available. A suitable pressure regulator must be provided to drop the cylinder pressure down to the ventilator's inlet pressure. Minute volume-divider-type ventilators can be entirely powered from the anaesthetic gas-mixture outlet of an anaesthetic machine.

When ventilation is only to involve air, many ventilators can be driven from an electric mains-powered compressor and they are sometimes provided with an optional rechargeable battery supply so that the ventilator can then be used in locations such as ambulances and aircraft.

8.10 Ventilator alarms

The provision of an inspiratory pressure alarm guards against the possibility of the ventilator attempting to try and inflate the room when the patient, perhaps restless, has become disconnected from the ventilator and the preset inflation pressure is not attained within a certain time. An expiratory tidal-volume alarm guards against the ventilator continuing to provide the full tidal volume, even though much of it is being lost through a leaky connection to the patient. A loss of power alarm guards against the loss of driving gas pressure or electrical power.

8.11 Bacterial decontamination of ventilators and tubing carrying respired gases

The hoses used with ventilators should be disinfected thoroughly after each use or be of a disposable variety. The channels of the ventilator through which respired gases pass should be easily and quickly removable for autoclaving or chemical sterilization as recommended by the manufacturer.

8.12 Infant ventilators

The high respiratory rate and small tidal volume of neonates requires that special purpose infant ventilators are used in special care baby units together with small lumen tracheostomy tubes and small face masks. A modern infant respirator of the continuous-flow, pressure-limited, time-cycled type might provide a range of inspiratory times from 0.1 to 2 seconds and a range of expiratory times from 0.2 to 30 seconds. Thus the highest ventilatory rate is 200 breaths per minute and the range of inspiratory flow rates available is 1 to 30 litres per minute. Some makes of adult ventilator incorporate a special group of settings for use with infants in terms of high ventilatory rates and small tidal volumes.

8.13 High frequency ventilation

This term is usually employed when the ventilatory frequency is more than four times the normal, e.g. 60–1800 breaths per minute (1 to 30 Hz). The tidal volume falls as the ventilatory rate is increased and the deadspace increases relative to the tidal volume which requires that high minute volumes are administered. Three techniques are in use: a) high frequency positive pressure ventilation (60–100 breaths per minute) via an endotracheal tube; b) high frequency jet ventilation (60–300 breaths per minute) with pulses of gas passed through a small bore cannula from a high pressure source of 1 to 4 atmospheres which may entrain additional gas. The tidal volumes employed are small and the airway pressures are low and spontaneous respiration is possible during ventilation. The tidal volumes involved are considerably less than the patient's anatomical deadspace, thus the movement of gas occurs by means of mechanisms other than the tidal exchange of gases; c) high frequency oscillation (3–30 Hz) by means of a sinewave pump.

The proposed advantages of high frequency oscillation include a reduction in the large swings of airway pressure produced by conventional ventilators and a decrease in the mean airway pressure. Care must be taken when using the technique since a high pressure source in the airway has the potential to produce significant trauma, and excessive inflation would result at large minute volumes if the exhaust circuit became occluded. At high minute volumes it is not easy to achieve an adequate humidification and the monitoring of airway pressure and lung volumes becomes difficult. However, high frequency ventilation is proving of value in surgery of the upper airways.

It has also been used for upper abdominal surgery: Babinski, M. F., Smith, R. B. and Sjostrand, U.H. (1985) 'Volume-controlled high frequency positive pressure ventilation for upper abdominal surgery', *Anaesthesia*, **40**, 619–23. In a comparison involving 74 patients undergoing biliary tract surgery, volume-controlled high frequency positive pressure ventilation was compared with intermittent positive pressure ventilation during anaesthesia. There were no statistically different differences in oxygenation or ventilation but significantly lower airway pressures and lower tidal volumes were recorded during the high frequency ventilation (ventilatory rate 60 per minute, constant inspiratory: expiratory ratio of 1: 3.5)

8.14 Humidifiers for use with ventilators

Patients who have to be ventilated for extended periods can become dehydrated when they are ventilated with dry air or a gas mixture. This causes a drying out of bronchial secretions which can lead to irritation and discomfort. The expirate from a patient is normally fully saturated with water vapour at body temperature as a result of the gases traversing the moist surfaces of the airways and lungs. This moistening mechanism copes when the patient is breathing room air but not with dry air over an extended period.

This loss of water can be replaced by the addition of water vapour to the inspired gas stream from an 'active' type of humidifier. This is often of the conventional 'bubbler' type in which the gas stream is bubbled through a temperature-controlled chamber containing sterile water. Wicks may be employed to provide a larger wet surface area over which the gas passes in order to provide a greater efficiency of water-vapour production.

A typical specification for a bubbler-type humidifier is that it should be able to deliver a gas stream with a minimum water-vapour content of 40 milligrams per litre (corresponding with a relative humidity of 90% at 37 degrees Celsius) over a volume-flow range of 6 to 10 litres per minute and allowing for peak flow rates of up to 30 litres per minute. The resistance to airflow should not exceed 1 cm of water at 10 litres per minute.

A new form of humidifier employs a humidity-exchange module consisting of approximately 200 water-vapour permeable hollow fibres. Water at a controlled temperature is passed around the outside of the fibres while the respired gases pass through the interior of the fibres. The large surface area of the fibres provides an efficient humidifier with a low compliance and an effective bacterial barrier between the water-supply reservoir and the inspired gases. There is a low condensation of liquid water and an automatic refill arrangement is provided based upon an optical sensor to detect the water level. The humidifier module can easily be exchanged and there is a digital display provided of the temperature of the inspired gas which can be adjusted in 0.5 degree Celsius increments over the range 0 to 38 degrees Celsius. Over the flow-rate range of 0 to 30 litres per minute, the relative humidity is greater than 95%.

Alternatively, scent-spray-type humidifiers are available in which a metered stream of sterile liquid water is pumped through a narrow orifice into the inspired gas stream where it vaporizes. Ultrasonic humidifiers produce cavitation in a chamber containing sterile water and the violent agitation of the water generates copious amounts of water vapour. Indeed with a powerful ultrasonic humidifier there can be a risk of drowning a patient due to an excess of water accumulating in the lungs unless the humidifier is used sparingly.

Bacteria can easily proliferate inside humidifiers. Only sterile water should be used and the interior of the humidifier regularly cleaned and sterilized in accordance with the manufacturer's instructions.

Electrically heated valves and hoses, with the heating powered from a low voltage supply, are often used to carry the humidified gas stream from humidifiers in order to prevent the condensation of liquid water which could interfere with the operation of moving parts.

In contrast, passive types of humidifier do not add additional water to the inspiratory circuit but merely conserve the water vapour which is present. In a typical construction, a copper gauze is mounted in a plastic holder designed to fit on to the exit of an endotracheal or tracheostomy tube. During expiration, water vapour at body temperature condenses on the room temperature metal gauze and is evaporated during the subsequent inspiration and fed back to the patient.

An alternative form of passive humidifier – a heat and moisture exchanger – consists of an outer plastic moulding, with a tube connection for attaching a supply of oxygen, which clips on to an inner plastic moulding sandwiching two pieces of the active element between them.

The active components comprise a hygroscopic and a bacteriostatic (chlorhexidine) material. The device has been designed for single use and is intended to be replaced daily or as necessary to prevent the accumulation of secretions from the patient. A 15 mm female connector allows for a direct connection to an endotracheal or tracheostomy tube. The resistance to gas flow is 10 pascals (1 mm water) at 30 litres per minute and the deadspace is 12 ml.

The moisture output is 23 mg per litre at room temperature for a 500 cc tidal volume at a rate of 10 breaths per minute and an inspiration/expiration ratio of 1:2. The moisture content of expired air fully saturated with water vapour at 34 degrees Celsius is 37.6 mg per litre.

8.15 Aerosol therapy

Devices which act to increase the water-vapour content of a gas stream are called humidifiers, whereas devices designed to generate aerosols are known as nebulizers (from 'nebula' meaning a cloud or mist). An aerosol is defined as a suspension of very fine particles, typically not more than 3 micrometres in diameter, with concentrations of 100 to 1000 particles per cubic centimetre of gas. The nasal filtering processes will completely remove particles greater than 5 micrometres in diameter, whereas those of 1 micrometre or less can pass the upper respiratory tract and are retained in pulmonary tissue. The pattern of ventilation in the upper tract influences the volume of particles reaching the alveoli, but does not influence particles of 1 micrometre or less once they have reached the alveoli. Slow, moderately deep breathing with breath holding at end-inspiration allows penetration of the alveoli by a signficiant number of particles and an adequate time interval for the smallest particles to diffuse into the alveoli and to settle by diffusion.

In a jet type of nebulizer, a stream of gas is arranged to enter the nebulizer chamber via a restricted orifice to provide a high velocity jet stream. The jet is directed across the top of a capillary tube; the lower end dips into the medication to be nebulized. The action of the jet is to produce a diminution in pressure at the top of the capillary tube so that liquid is forced up the capillary. As it reaches the top of the tube it is continuously blown away by the gas stream as a series of small particles and is arranged to strike one or more baffles (barriers). These further fragment the particles and groups of particles which coalesce drop out of the stream of gas, which emerges containing particles of the correct therapeutic size for inhalation by the patient. The medication may often be a bronchodilator or mucolytic agent. Anti-spasm drugs can be administered in aerosol form for the symptomatic therapy of asthmatic conditions.

8.16 'Intelligent' ventilator systems

Technology has improved the design of mechanical ventilators to an extent that the most modern are microprocessor-controlled and are provided with at least one communication port for connection to a computer network. It has been estimated that up to 8 megabytes of ventilator-derived data can be collected per patient per day. This large increase in the volume of data, and the interrelationships between the data items, creates problems of information management. If these results available from more powerful technology are to be employed to the best clinical effect, there is a need to enhance the capability of the ventilator by converting data into information and ultimately transferring this into knowledge. This needs to be in a form readily usable by doctors and nurses and of value to the management of the patient's condition. The branch of science which deals with the incorporation of a knowledge component into instrumentation is known as 'artificial intelligence'. When machines exhibit some form of intelligence, the computer software which controls the reasoning strategy is usually termed a 'knowledge-based system' (KBS).

Integration of ventilator data with other key data items, for example, blood-gas and pH data, requires a KBS which models complex interrelationships in a similar fashion to the reasoning of an experienced clinician who evaluates the condition of a patient by analysing all the available data. These data relationships form what is known as a 'knowledge model of the domain' and are elicited from expert clinicians in the management of patients on ventilators. As the KBS must be able to reason about any decision which it makes, the system must include provision for the supply of explanations. These why? or how? queries can be generated by simply tracing and analysing the computer-based reasoning process. The explanation facility is an important element of a KBS, as it allows the user to check the validity of any decision. Carson, E. R., Chelsom, J. J. L. and Summers, R. (1990) 'Progress with measurement, information and decision-making in critical care medicine', *Measurement*, **9**, 104–10, detail advances in knowledge-based technology applied to the high dependency environment. For ventilator therapy there is a need to minimize the difference between the chosen settings of the ventilator and the needs of the patient. Carson *et al.* suggest that the development of a KBS will aid the clinical decision-maker.

Sittig, D. F. (1987) 'Computerised management of patient care in a complex controlled clinical trial in the Intensive Care Unit' in *Proceedings of the 11th Annual Symposium on Computer Applications*, (ed.) W. W. Stead, New York: Institution of Electrical and Electronic Engineers, 225–32, shows that in a controlled clinical trial (without computer-based decision support) the correct therapeutic action was taken for 85% of patients with hypoxaemia, but the remaining 15% were at risk of a life-threatening event

Figure 8.5 Block diagram of an
Intelligent Ventilator system.

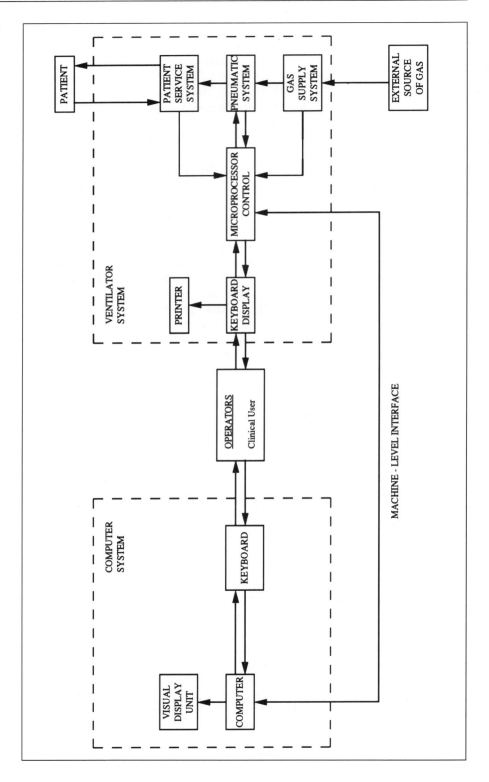

for an unacceptable period of time, sometimes in excess of one hour after the initial therapeutic action. There is thus a benefit to be obtained from the introduction of decision support in automatic ventilation of the lungs.

Summers, R. (1990) 'Advances in intelligent instrumentation for the management of the critically ill patient' *Measurement and Control*, **23**, 263–6, describes an intelligent ventilator. The basic description of the system is shown in Figure 8.5 where the patient, ventilator, KBS resident in the computer and the clinical users are depicted. Note: the ventilator has a communication port which connects it with the associated computer.

Knowledge-based decision support is particularly required when weaning the patient off the ventilator. A conceptual model of the weaning

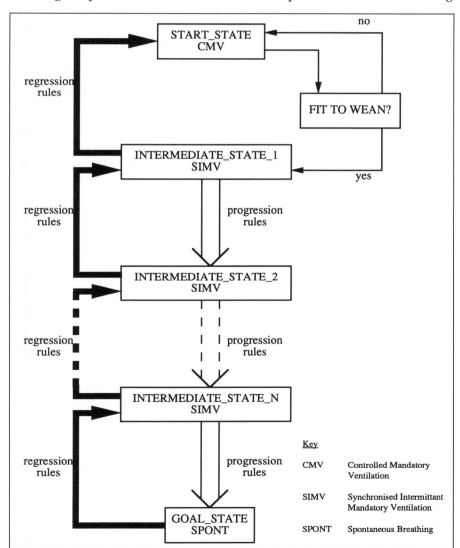

Figure 8.6 Conceptual model of the weaning process.

process is shown in Figure 8.6 and indicates the three types of rules required. The 'fit-to-wean' rule set is invoked when weaning commences and tests to see if an extensive set of qualifying conditions have been met to ensure that other physiological systems are stable. The patient continues the weaning process, but checks are made on progress and, if necessary, the patient can revert to a previous set of ventilatory variables using the regression rule set. Both progression and regression rules use blood-gas data as a means of determining the progression of the patient along predetermined paths. The regression rule set also uses the patient's respiratory pattern as an indicant of his clinical status.

Rules can be generated directly from the conceptual model of the weaning process, Figure 8.7. The inclusion of a meta-rule (a rule which acts on other rules) allows the system to err on the side of safety in the unlikely occurrence of progression and regression rules succeeding simultaneously: that is, the patient will then revert to the previous state.

The actual rules contained in a practical knowledge base and the reasoning strategy adopted are a little more complex than those presented so far. To give an indication of what is involved in the implementation of an intelligent ventilator system when dealing with the weaning of patients from intermittent positive pressure ventilation, consider the knowledge rules of the 'GANESH' system of Dojat, M., Brochard, L., Lemaire, F. and Harf, A. (1992) "A knowledge-based system for assisted ventilation of patients in intensive care units', *International Journal of Clinical Monitoring and Computing*, **9**, 239–50. The knowledge required by the system is represented in the form of 'production rules' which in their simplest form comprise:

IF   condition(s)
THEN   action(s)

Figure 8.7 Knowledge rules derived from the conceptual model of the weaning process.

WEANING_RULE_1 :   IF START_STATE
                    and fit_to_wean
                    THEN go to INTERMEDIATE_STATE_1.

PROGRESSSION_RULE_2 :   IF INTERMEDIATE_STATE_N
                         and progression_rules_succeed
                         THEN go to INTERMEDIATE_STATE_N+1.

REGRESSSION_RULE_3 :   IF INTERMEDIATE_STATE_N
                        and regression_rules_succeed
                        THEN go to INTERMEDIATE_STATE_N–1.

TERMINATION_RULE_4 :   IF GOAL_STATE
                        THEN STOP.

META_RULE_1 :   If regression conditions succeed
                 and progression conditions succeed
                 THEN do REGRESSION_RULE_3.

More complicated production rules can be constructed by using an 'AND' or an 'OR' to link conditions or actions together. Some examples of the GANESH rule-base which include these more complicated rules are:

Rule 1 IF the patient is tracheotomized
   THEN pressure-supported ventilation (PSV) before weaning can be envisaged at 5 cm water.

Rule 2 IF pressure support is equal to or greater than 15 cm water
   AND pressure support does not exceed 20 cm water
   THEN period of observation should be 4 hours.

Rule 3 IF the tidal volume is less than the pre-determined minimum
   OR the end-tidal carbon dioxide tension exceeds 7.32 kPa (55 mm mercury)
   THEN the ventilation is 'insufficient'.

Rule 4 IF the respiration is 'tachypneaic'
   OR the ventilation is 'insufficient'
   AND the previous respiratory state is 'normal'
   THEN the stability of the patient's respiratory condition is 'bad'.

Rule 5 IF the patient's respiratory condition is 'bad'
   THEN increase the pressure support by 4 cm water
   AND review the situation after 5 minutes.

Rule 6 IF the minute volume is low i.e. hypoventilation
   THEN raise alarm (level 4)
   AND switch to mechanical ventilation.

These production rules can be interpreted as follows:

Rule 1 infers information from data entered by the user of the system and indicates that a pressure-support value of 5 cm water is necessary before weaning can commence.

Rule 2 assesses the patient's respiratory state and indicates a 'window' of acceptable values for pressure support and the length of time for which the patient should remain within these limits before the pressure support can be reduced, i.e. if the pressure support required is in the range 15 to 20 cm water, this level of support should be provided for 4 hours.

Rule 3 provides two conditions against which the patient's respiration can be judged to be inadequate.

Rule 4 provides an indication of the patient's progress towards adequate respiration. In the example given, the patient's respiratory status is deteriorating and assistance needs to be provided promptly. Rule 4 indicates the presence of a problem and Rule 5 provides information on the corrective action. It can be seen that the rules of the knowledge-base chain together, yielding the system's strategy of reasoning. The respiratory stability of the patient is reported as 'bad' in the action portion of Rule 4.

This causes Rule 5 to operate because its condition portion matches the requirement for action. As a consequence, pressure support is raised by an additional 4 cm water and a further review of the patient's progress is requested at 5 minute intervals.

Rule 6 is an example of a rule which sounds an alarm. If the patient is not respiring adequately then alarm 4 is activated (a coded version for that particular type of alarm signal). A need to put the patient on to automatic ventilation of the lungs is also indicated.

The complete GANESH system comprises 142 production rules and is dependent on the use of an infra-red gas analyser to obtain the end-tidal carbon dioxide tension values.

Blood-gas and pH analysers, pulse oximeters and renal dialysis

9

9.1 Introduction

In the management of high dependency patients a knowledge of the blood pH together with the tensions (partial pressures) of oxygen and carbon dioxide in arterial blood is important, when circulation or respiration is impaired and there are associated metabolic disorders. The development of specific electrode systems for these variables has made possible routine estimations on small volume blood samples, e.g. for neonates. Direct, invasive measurements with blood samples are the most accurate but transcutaneous devices for the indirect monitoring of blood-gas tensions and of oxygen saturation are now in common use.

Blood-gas and blood pH measurements can be required at any hour of the day or night at short notice. It is essential that the blood-gas analyser should always be available at the correct operating temperature (normally 37 degrees Celsius) in a fully functioning and calibrated state. The self-checking and calibrating facilities of modern analysers help substantially in these respects. It is equally important that the staff concerned should have been trained in its use and that the blood samples are correctly labelled and the presence of air bubbles in the samples has been avoided. Syringes should be tightly capped to prevent the loss of high gas tensions to the atmosphere and all syringes used must be clean and an anti-coagulant employed. The syringes containing blood samples should be stored on ice to minimize metabolic changes occurring in the blood-gas tensions if there is a delay before the samples can be analysed.

Fully automated microcomputer-controlled blood-gas and pH analysers contain three sets of active electrodes (for pH, oxygen and carbon dioxide tensions) all of which operate with a common cuvette containing a blood sample which may have a volume of only 240 microlitres. Each active electrode works in conjunction with its own stable reference electrode against which its output is measured. The pH and carbon dioxide electrode pairs generate a voltage output and the polarographic oxygen electrode pair generates a current output. The electrodes and cuvette are temperature controlled. Each electrode system needs calibrating, the pH system against buffer solutions of known pH values and the oxygen and carbon dioxide systems against known gas mixtures or tonometered whole blood.

Three additional ion selective electrodes can be provided to allow the measurement of sodium, potassium, chloride or ionized calcium concentrations using the same 240 microlitre blood sample as for blood-gas and pH determinations. Variables such as blood base excess, actual bicarbonate and standard bicarbonate, total dissolved carbon dioxide, calculated oxygen saturation, alveolar-arterial oxygen difference, anion gap and respiratory index can be calculated, Figure 9.1.

9.2 The definition of pH and normal values for human blood

Pondus Hydrogens (pH) – the concentration of hydrogen ions – was proposed by Sorenson in 1909. He defined pH as the negative logarithm of the hydrogen ion concentration of the solution of interest, i.e. $pH = -\log (H^+)$, so that a pH range of 0 to 14 covers a range of hydrogen ion concentrations from 1 to 10 raised to the power -14. Normal values for human whole blood at 37 degrees Celsius are 7.35 to 7.45 for arterial blood and

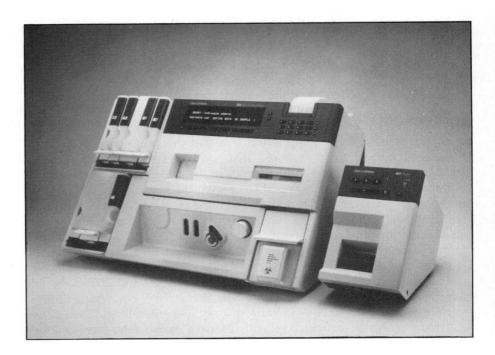

Figure 9.1 Ciba-Corning Model 288 blood-gas system provides direct readings of blood pH, pCO_2, pO_2, Na and K together with a choice of Ca or Cl. (Courtesy Ciba Corning Diagnostics Ltd.)

7.32 to 7.42 for venous blood. The concentration of hydrogen ions in blood is often quoted in terms of nanomoles per litre. Thus a pH of 6.90 is equivalent to a hydrogen ion concentration of antilog (–6.90) = 1.25 × 10 to the power –7 moles per litre, i.e. 125 nanomoles per litre.

9.3 The pH glass electrode-reference electrode system

The lower end of a pH sensitive glass electrode is fabricated from a special thin pH sensitive glass, Figure 9.2. The interior of the hollow electrode contains a buffer solution of a known and stable pH value into which dips a chlorided silver wire leading out through a glass-to-metal seal at the top of the electrode, to connect via a well-insulated cable to one input terminal of the pH meter. The bottom end of the electrode is in contact with the blood sample whose pH is to be measured. The sample occupies a cuvette into which are placed three separate electrodes for blood pH, carbon dioxide and oxygen tensions. The tensions are the partial pressures of the gases in blood. The reference electrode, Figure 9.3, is joined to the cuvette via a 'salt bridge' of saturated potassium chloride solution. Its electrical output is connected to the other input terminal of the pH meter.

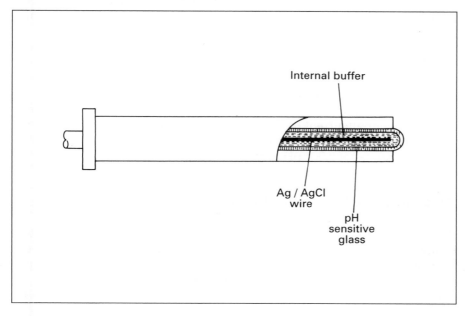

Internal buffer

Ag / AgCl
wire

pH
sensitive
glass

Figure 9.2 Cutaway view of a glass pH electrode. (Courtesy Instrumentation Laboratory Ltd.)

The pH sensitive glass is permeable to hydrogen ions in the blood sample and when an equilibrium has been established between the rate of diffusion of hydrogen ions across the glass membrane in either direction, a d.c. voltage is developed between the inside and outside surface of the glass. This voltage is proportional to the difference between the pH values of the stable pH (buffer) solution inside the glass electrode and the pH of the blood sample. A pH glass electrode in good condition has a sensitivity

Figure 9.3 Calomel reference electrode. (Courtesy Instrumentation Laboratory Ltd.)

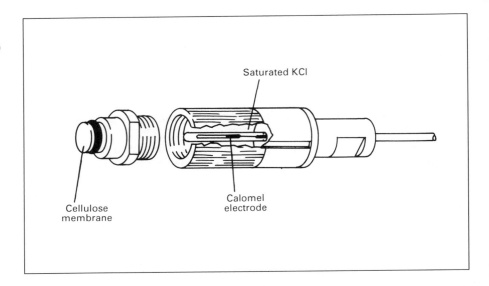

Figure 9.3 Calomel reference electrode. (Courtesy Instrumentation Laboratory Ltd.)

of approximately 60 millivolts per pH unit change. If it falls significantly below this value the electrode will need to be refurbished or changed. The sensitivity is temperature dependent and hence the sample cuvette and all the electrodes should be thermostatted at a temperature which is usually 37 degrees Celsius plus or minus 0.1 degrees Celsius.

The glass electrode-reference electrode combination behaves as a battery whose electromotive force (EMF) – open circuit voltage – is pH dependent. Its internal resistance is high, of the order of 100 megohms or more, so that the associated pH meter must be an electrometer type of millivolt-meter with an input resistance of at least 100 000 megohms so that it draws a negligible input current from the high resistance cell. A typical range for a blood pH meter would be 6.000 to 8.000 pH units and it must be possible to detect changes of 0.001 pH units (60 microvolts).

9.4 Buffer solutions for the calibration of blood pH meters

A pH meter must always be calibrated before it is used by allowing it to sample two buffer solutions of accurately known pH values and setting the controls of the meter to read correctly on these values. Typical calibration-buffer solutions would have values of 6.840 and 7.384 pH units at 37 degrees Celsius. Buffer solutions are expensive to purchase and must be handled with care to avoid dilution or contamination.

9.5 The carbon dioxide electrode

Hypercarbia, although not as dangerous as hypoxaemia, can lead to the production of cardiac arrhythmias, and the management of patients on ventilators should be aimed at maintaining blood-gas and pH values within normal values. A normal range for arterial carbon dioxide tension is 4.7 to 6.0 kPa (35–45 mm Hg). Both oxygen and carbon dioxide tensions are now usually quoted in terms of kilopascals, but blood-gas analysers can provide an alternative scaling in millimetres of mercury. The direct reading carbon dioxide tension electrode, Figure 9.4, has greatly facilitated the monitoring of carbon dioxide tensions: Severinghaus, J. W. and Bradley, A. F. (1958) 'Electrodes for PO_2 and PCO_2 determination', *Journal of Applied Physiology*, **13**, 515. Basically this sensor consists of a pH glass electrode which has a thin layer of sodium bicarbonate solution held between the front face of the glass membrane and a thin silicone rubber membrane. The function of the membrane is to allow carbon dioxide gas from the blood to diffuse through its pores into the bicarbonate solution. Proteinaceous material in the blood which would clog up the pH sensitive glass cannot penetrate the membrane and 'poison' the electrode.

In a practical electrode arrangement, the sodium bicarbonate solution is localized within the pores of an inert nylon mesh placed under the outer Teflon (polytetrafluoroethylene) membrane which is permeable to carbon dioxide molecules. Both the nylon mesh and the membrane are held in place on the cylindrical body of the electrode by means of O-rings.

The change in pH of the bicarbonate solution as a result of the addition of carbon dioxide is logarithmically related to the blood carbon dioxide

Figure 9.4 Carbon dioxide electrode. (Courtesy Instrumentation Laboratory Ltd.)

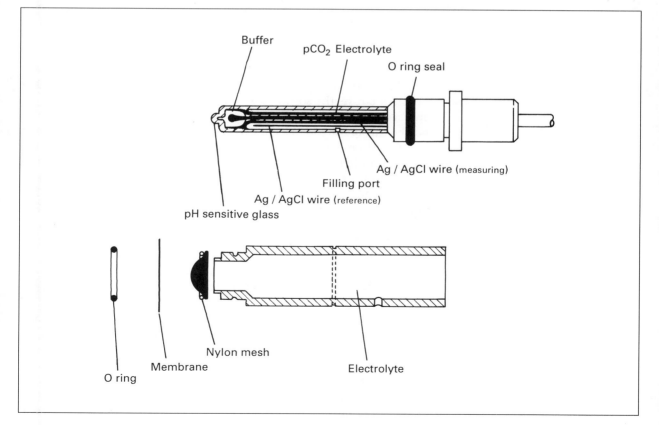

tension. An amplifier having an anti-logarithmically related gain characteristic is employed to produce a linear relationship between the pH change and carbon dioxide tension which can be scaled in kilopascals or millimetres of mercury. A typical range would be 0.7 to 33.3 kPa (5 to 250 mmHg).

A 10-fold increase in carbon dioxide tension is approximately equivalent to a reduction of one pH unit, as the effect of the carbon dioxide is to render the solution more acidic. The carbon dioxide electrode is used in conjunction with a silver/silver chloride reference electrode and the combination is thermostatted as for a glass pH electrode.

9.6 The calibration of a carbon dioxide electrode

The most accurate method is to utilize blood tonometered in a thin film tonometer (Chalmers, C., Bird, B. D. and Whitwam, J. G. (1974) 'Evaluation of a new thin film tonometer', *British Journal of Anaesthesia*, **46**, 253–9) in turn with two gas mixtures, each having a known carbon dioxide partial pressure. In a blood-gas analyser the gas mixtures are passed in turn through a heat exchanger and humidifier to ensure that they are fully saturated with water vapour and at 37 degrees Celsius. They then enter the sample cuvette. Suppose that one of the gas mixtures contains 5% by volume of carbon dioxide. The barometric pressure is B mmHg and the saturated vapour pressure of water at 37 degrees Celsius is 47 mmHg. The partial pressure of carbon dioxide in the gas mixture is given by $(5/100)(B–47)$ mmHg. To convert to kilopascals, use the factor 1 mmHg = 0.133 kPa. The use of a tonometer removes the possibility that the electrode might read differently for a gas mixture alone and with blood equilibrated with the gas mixture, the so-called blood-gas difference.

In practice the blood-gas difference for modern electrodes is insignificant and the carbon dioxide electrode can be calibrated against two known gas mixtures. Both are required to adjust the balance and slope of the linear calibration line. The balance control is used to set the instrument to read correctly on the first mixture and the slope control to make it read correctly on the second mixture, thus defining the calibration line. Another possibility is the use of commercially available quality-control solutions comprising a tonometered buffer solution with known pH, carbon dioxide and oxygen tensions often packaged in a 1 ml ampoule.

9.7 The polarographic oxygen electrode

A deficiency of oxygen can be crucially important in the management of a patient and the availability of direct reading oxygen electrodes has been a major step forward. The polarographic oxygen electrode, Figure 9.5, is a current generating system in contrast to the voltage generating pH and carbon dioxide tension electrodes: Clark, L. C. Jnr., (1956) 'Monitor and control of blood and tissue oxygen tensions', *Transactions of the American Society of Artificial Internal Organs*, **2**, 41. In the case of the oxygen electrode

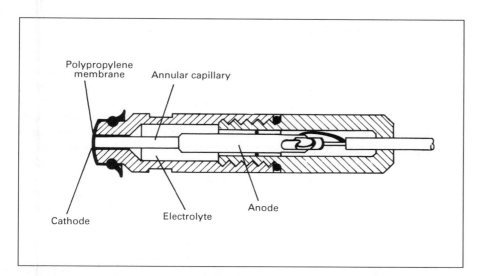

Figure 9.5 Polagraphic oxygen electrode. (Courtesy Instrumentation Laboratory Ltd.)

a d.c. polarizing voltage of 0.6 V from a stable battery is applied across a combination of a silver/silver chloride reference electrode and a platinum cathode which is covered with a polypropylene membrane. The platinum wire has its bottom end ground flush with the glass sheath to which it is fused. The membrane-covered wire cathode faces into the sample cuvette. The sample is also connected to the reference electrode by means of a salt bridge.

Oxygen molecules in the blood sample diffuse to the cathode via the porous membrane where the oxygen is reduced, each oxygen molecule reaching the cathode reacting with four electrons. The resulting small current (nanoamperes) is measured by means of a sensitive current amplifier. The final output display can be in the form of an analogue meter reading but is more usually a digital display scaled in terms of oxygen tension in kilopascals or millimetres of mercury. A typical range would be 0 to 212.8 kPa (0–1600 mmHg). The normal range for arterial oxygen tension is 9.2–15.4 kPa (69–116 mmHg). The three individual electrodes for pH, carbon dioxide and oxygen tensions share a common sample cuvette and are all thermostatted together with their reference electrodes in a water bath or a heated metal block.

9.8 The calibration of an oxygen electrode

The use of tonometered blood with a known oxygen tension represents the most accurate technique, but in practice, warmed and humidified known gas mixtures are employed to calibrate both the oxygen and carbon dioxide electrodes. Typical calibration gas mixtures might be (10% carbon dioxide and 90% nitrogen) and (5% carbon dioxide, 12% oxygen, 83% nitrogen). Commercial tonometered buffer solutions with known pH, oxygen and carbon dioxide tensions contained in sealed ampoules can also be used for quick quality-control checks.

9.9 Conventional blood-gas analysers

Modern blood-gas analysers are controlled by an integrated micro-processor and are designed to be as foolproof and automatic as possible so that they can be relied upon for use on a 24-hour basis. They can be calibrated on a one- or two-point basis on command by the operator, if present, or automatically on a preset time schedule. Derived variables such as standard and total bicarbonate and percentage oxygen saturation can be calculated on command and a hard copy printed of all the results together with the patient identification details, the time and date.

The software provided to operate a blood-gas analyser may require that the operator enters a personal identification number (PIN) before the analyser will operate or reveal previously stored results in order to preserve confidentiality of patient data.

Evaluation Report MDD/92/45 'IL BGE 1400 Blood Gas Analyser' by the Medical Devices Directorate of the United Kingdom's Department of Health comments on the development of 'biochemistry profile' analysers capable of measuring pH, PO_2, PCO_2, sodium, potassium, chloride, glucose, ionized calcium, haematocrit and lactate. Advances in ion selective electrodes have allowed for the measurement of sodium, potassium, chloride and ionized calcium from the same blood sample of 240 microlitres used for the blood-gas measurement (Vadgama, P. and Alberti, K. G. (1985) 'Bedside monitoring: the role of electrodes' in *Recent Advances in Clinical Biochemistry*, **3**, 255–72). This type of comprehensive analyser is finding a place in intensive care, coronary care and special care baby units, operating rooms and satellite laboratories. It is important that an anti-coagulant is used with the blood sample to prevent blood clotting in the heated interior of the analyser. Lithium heparin at a final concentration of less than 15 international units per ml or sodium, potassium and calcium balanced lithium heparin at a final heparin concentration of 25–50 international units per ml is recommended for blood-gas and electrolyte analysis in the Evaluation Report MDD/92/45 of September 1992 from the Medical Devices Directorate of the United Kingdom's Department of Health. Mann, S. W. and Green, A. (1986) 'Interference from heparin in commercial heparinized tubes in the measurement of plasma sodium by ion selective electrode: a note of caution', *Annals of Clinical Biochemistry*, **23**, 355–6, report that high concentrations of heparin can reduce the measured sodium activity.

9.10 Computer support of blood-gas and pH data

Most modern blood-gas analysers are provided with a communication port which enables the transfer of data from the analyser to either a dedicated computer or to a computer network where the data becomes more widely available. The trend in the design of blood-gas analysers is not only to provide data-processing (for example, to calculate the standard bicarbonate) but also for data interpretation. Thus, the field of blood-gas analysis is another example of where an element of machine intelligence has been added to the instrumentation system. Computer programs which use simple algorithms for interpreting acid-base findings have been available since the 1960s. Gradually, these programs have become more sophisticated and can now propose a tentative diagnosis and therapy for even triple acid-base disorders without much difficulty.

9.11 Computer interpretation of acid-base disorders: a case study

It might be queried as to why there has been so much research activity in what some could describe as a relatively trivial exercise. Evidence from several studies shows that whereas specialists find the interpretation of blood-gas results straightforward, it is an area which is extremely confusing for non-specialists such as new entrants to intensive care nursing and junior medical staff. The following three examples are indicative of the literature in this growth area.

Hingston, D. N., Irwin, R. S., Pratter, M. R. and Dalen, J. E. (1982) 'A computerised interpretation of arterial pH and blood-gas data: do physicians need it?', *Respiratory Care*, **27**, 809–15 reported that 71% of clinicians contacted in their study did not think they needed computer assistance, although only 39% of the acid-base disturbances were diagnosed correctly when the same group was tested without computer support.

Schreck, D. M., Zacherias, D. and Grunau, C. F. (1986) 'Diagnosis of complex acid-base disorders: physician performance versus the microcomputer', *Annals of Emergency Medicine*, **15**, 164–70 showed that a cross-section of clinicians had an 86% success rate in diagnosing single acid-base disoders; a 49% success rate in diagnosing a double acid-base disorder and only a 17% success rate in diagnosing triple acid-base disorders.

Broughton, J. O. and Kennedy, T. C. (1984) 'Interpretation of arterial blood-gases by computer', *Chest*, **85**, 148–9 reveal that 'a drop in untimely or inappropriate therapeutic responses' from 33% to 9% was achieved when the clinicians were assisted by a computer-based interpretation system.

Much of the emphasis of current research in this area is concentrated on data (or information) integration. If a blood-gas analyser is connected to a computer network, the interpreted blood-gas data form one part of a patient data-management system (see Chapter 7). Kazda, A., Jabor, A., Zamencik, M. and Masek, K. (1989) 'Monitoring acid-base electrolyte disturbances in intensive care', *Advances in Clinical Chemistry*, **27**, 201–68 suggest that information obtained from blood-gas analysers can be exploited in an optimal way only if there is a simultaneous evaluation of the patient's medical history, clinical state and laboratory findings. This approach is facilitated by the use of patient data-management systems.

The Puritan-Bennett Corporation market a real-time intra-arterial blood-gas analyser (Model PB 3300). An attractive possibility may be to connect the output from this analyser to a ventilator as part of a closed-loop system to control the patient's blood-gas concentrations. In such a system, the patient-management strategy depends upon a combination of blood-gas, ventilator derived and other data which allow the settings of the ventilator to be automatically adjusted. Before this type of arrangement can be accepted into routine clinical practice, it must be thoroughly tested in order that safety considerations can be properly investigated and implemented.

It is evident that computer-assisted decision-making is developing in areas such as fluid balance and ventilator management as an important adjunct to doctors and nurses responsible for intensive care. Indeed, completion of the control loop to produce life-support systems which are computer controlled subject to instructions from clinical staff is leading to experimental systems which are providing valuable experience. However, these developments have to be sustained against a background of solid clinical experience on behalf of the staff concerned.

Blood-gas analysers are often provided with a comprehensive data-management system, typically utilizing two floppy disk drives – one for the system disk and the other for the data disk. The system disk holds the operational software and can also hold quality-control data sufficient for at least one year's operation with the facility to assay each of three values of quality control material up to 12 times per day. The data for the pH, PCO_2 and PO_2 channels can be recalled and plotted for a given month or operator. Values falling outside the known ranges for the quality-control material will be flagged up. The data disk can typically hold 6300 results from up to 630 patients whose identifications have been entered into the analyser. The storage, retrieval and print-out of results is governed by the use of operator identification numbers. Calibration of a blood-gas/electrolyte analyser typically requires the use of two buffer solutions providing known values of pH, sodium, potassium and ionized calcium and two known gas mixtures of carbon dioxide and oxygen.

Data from a blood-gas analyser can be interpreted automatically by means of a computer program and used to identify (diagnose) acid-base disorders. These can be classified into 'simple' disorders or more complex 'mixed' disorders where more than one simple disorder occurs in a patient at the same time. The data set used for this task comprises the patient's pH, arterial carbon dioxide tension, bicarbonate, base excess and anion gap, all of which are obtainable from a modern blood-gas analyser.

9.11.1 Interpretation of simple acid-base disorders

There are four simple acid-base disorders. Respiratory acidosis and respiratory alkalosis in which the retention or depletion of carbon dioxide is responsible for the change in blood pH value. In metabolic acidosis and metabolic alkalosis it is the retention or depletion of bicarbonate which causes a change in pH.

Respiratory acidosis and respiratory alkalosis are produced by a single physiological process: that is, by an abnormal pattern of respiration. This is the direct cause of the imbalance in carbon dioxide. Metabolic disturbances are more complex. As an example, consider the following three causes of metabolic acidosis:

1   A loss of body alkali which causes the plasma bicarbonate level to fall.
2   An increase in the production of normal body acids which will eventually overwhelm the renal excretory mechanism.
3   An impaired renal excretory mechanism. This will cause an increase in the level of body acids (assuming that production is unaffected).

In the first case, lost bicarbonate ions (alkaline) are replaced by chloride ions (also alkaline) so that the anion gap remains within the normal range. A metabolic acidosis caused by a loss of body alkali is therefore termed a normal anion gap (NAG) metabolic acidosis. In cases 2) and 3) the bicarbonate ions are replaced by naturally occurring substances such as lactate, phosphate and sulphate. The anion gap is raised causing a so-called high anion gap (HAG) metabolic acidosis. Figure 9.6 illustrates the classification of simple disorders, showing the corresponding values expected for each item of data (L = Low; N = Normal; H = High). Where two possible values are given, either value is possible for the given disorder.

The body has its own homeostatic mechanism, termed a compensatory response, which acts when the blood pH is either raised or lowered due to an outside influence. Metabolic acid-base disorders are compensated by means of an appropriate increase or decrease in ventilation, whereas respiratory disturbances are compensated by some form of metabolic action. A further complexity superimposed upon the compensatory response is its time course of action. The compensatory response for metabolic disturbances is almost immediate as the pattern of spontaneous respiration can be changed at will. However, compensation for respiratory acid-base imbalances takes a far longer period of time as changes in metabolism are dependent on a number of variables such as renal function. Hence, it is possible to classify respiratory acid-base disturbances into acute and chronic disorders: in the former there is no apparent metabolic compensation (less than 12 to 14 hours); in the latter, a compensatory response can be detected.

9.11.2 The interpretation of mixed acid-base disorders

Mixed disorders of acid-base metabolism occur when two or more of the simple disorders are present in the patient concurrently. This type of disorder can be detected when the expected compensatory response of a simple-acid-base disturbance is not evident. It follows that it is not possible to have a mixed respiratory acidosis and respiratory alkalosis because carbon dioxide depletion and retention are mutually exclusive events. However, either respiratory disorder can occur with one or more metabolic disturbances (giving rise to mixed and triple disorders respectively) and any combination of metabolic alkalosis with a NAG or HAG metabolic acidosis can also occur. A summary of the types of mixed acid-base

Figure 9.6 Classification of data values for simple acid-base disorders. (Courtesy J.J.L. Chelsom.)

DISORDER	pH	PaCO$_2$	HCO$_3^-$	BE	AG
Acute respiratory acidosis	L	H	N, H	N	N
Chronic respiratory acidosis	N, L	H	H	H	N
Acute respiratory alkalosis	H	L	N, L	N	N, H
Chronic respiratory alkalosis	N, H	L	L	L	N
Metabolic alkalosis	H	N	H	H	H, N
Compensated metabolic alkalosis	N, H	H	H	H	N
HAG metabolic acidosis	L	N	L	L	H
Compensated HAG metabolic acidosis	N, L	L	L	L	H
NAG metabolic acidosis	L	N	L	L	N
Compensated NAG metabolic acidosis	N, L	L	L	L	N

disorder possible is shown in Figure 9.7. For simplication, in Figure 9.7 the condition shown as 'mixed metabolic acidosis' could be any combination of HAG- or NAG-based disorders. Similarly, where the term metabolic acidosis is used to describe one element of the disorder, it can be HAG or NAG or a mixed metabolic acidosis. Finally, where a respiratory disturbance is indicated, it could be either chronic or acute.

9.11.3 Implementation details

The computer-based approach to the interpretation of pathology-laboratory data, including acid-base disorders, described here has been developed over a number of years within the Department of Systems Science of the City University in London. The approach adopted uses a dual perspective of the clinical problem. Identification of the clinical problem – identification from available data on acid-base disorders, hypoxaemia and respiratory failure which may provide a sufficient indication for the commencement of appropriate therapy; and diagnosis of the underlying disease processes which are responsible for yielding the measured set of data. This dual perspective mimics the actions of clinicians

DISORDER	pH	PaCO$_2$	HCO$_3^-$	BE	AG
Mixed metabolic acidosis	L	L	L	L	H, N
Respiratory alkalosis + metabolic alkalosis	H	L, N	H, N	H, N	H
Respiratory acidosis + metabolic acidosis	L	H, N	L, N	L	H
Respiratory acidosis + metabolic alkalosis	N	H	H	H	N
Respiratory alkalosis + metabolic acidosis	N	L	L	L	H, N
Metabolic alkalosis + metabolic acidosis	N	----	variable	----	H, N
Metabolic alkalosis + metabolic acidosis + respiratory acidosis	L	----	variable	----	H, N
Metabolic alkalosis + metabolic acidosis + respiratory akalosis	H	----	variable	----	H, N

Figure 9.7 Classification of data values for mixed acid-base disorders. (Courtesy J.J.L. Chelsom.)

since they often produce a working diagnosis based on patient history, signs and symptoms. Blood-gas analysis usually provides confirmatory information regarding diagnosis of the patient's problem. If the results are inconsistent with the working diagnosis, then the diagnosis must be revised or another blood-gas sample should be taken and the reasoning process repeated. The program can be run on a laptop computer.

These two views are reflected in Figure 9.8 which shows the physiological diagnosis of acid-base disorders based on data available from blood-gas analyses (lower panel) and a clinical diagnosis based on a clinician's working diagnosis (upper panel). Each panel is split into a number of levels and the elements which act on the data in some way are termed 'knowledge sources'. At the start of computer assistance, the user enters the working diagnosis for the patient concerned together with the blood-gas values. The lower panel produces a differential diagnosis of disorders and this is matched with the working diagnosis in order that a critique of the clinician's decision-making process can be obtained.

The 'physiological'diagnosis panel comprises four distinct levels: 'raw data', 'processed data', 'hypotheses' and 'diagnosis'. Data from a database of clinical findings, including blood-gas results, are written to the 'raw data' level by the 'write data' knowledge source. The 'data derivation' knowledge source monitors what is input at this level and if further data

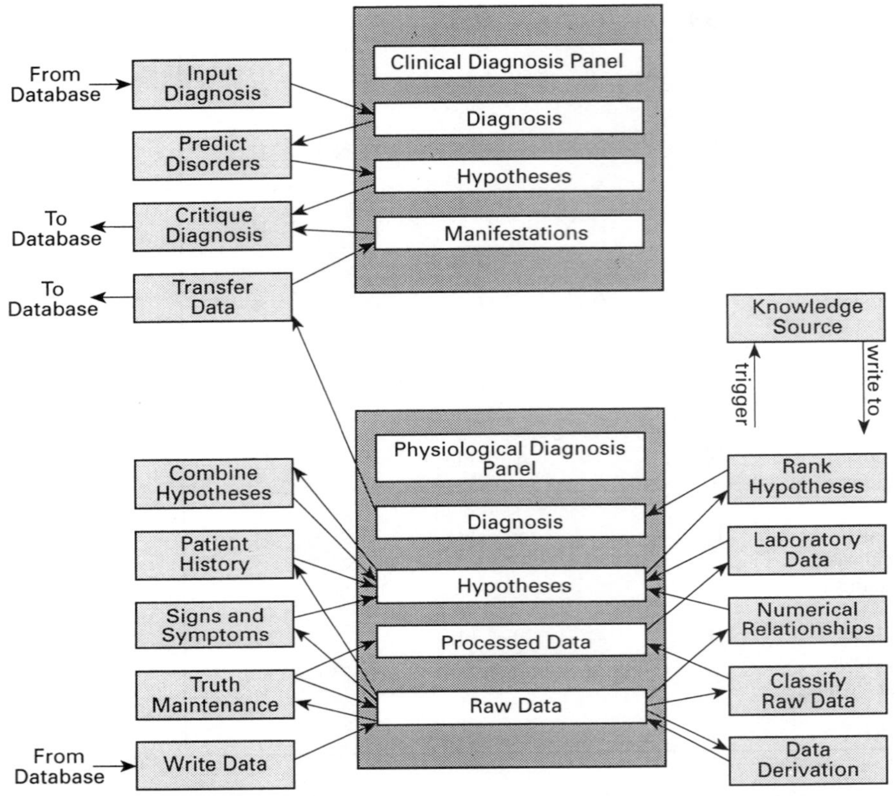

Figure 9.8 Dual-panel implementation of a system for pathology laboratory data interpretation. (Courtesy J.J.L. Chelsom.)

can be derived from the data already entered, these are added to the 'raw data' level. If the user wants to change any of the measured values (perhaps to remove artifact) at the 'raw data' level, the 'truth maintenance' knowledge source is activated. Altering the data at the lowest level ensures that any changes made are propagated throughout the system. The raw data is then classified by the 'classify raw data' knowledge source, the results being transferred to the 'processed data' level of the physiological diagnosis panel. This knowledge source changes numerical data into qualitative descriptors, e.g. instead of numbers representing the value of an item of data, the terms 'high', 'normal' or 'low' are used before any further processing is attempted.

Four evidence handling knowledge sources – 'numerical relationships', 'signs and symptoms', 'laboratory data' and 'patient history' – are used to formulate hypotheses of physiological disorders. For example, the 'laboratory data' knowledge source uses Tables as shown in Figures 9.6 and 9.7. The system also contains details of associational links between clinical observations and disorders. These are organized into a taxonomy and form the basis of the three evidence handling knowledge sources.

At the hypothesis level of the physiological diagnosis panel, several hypotheses are usually generated for each set of data entered. These multiple hypotheses are aggregated by the 'combine hypotheses' knowledge source, allowing only a single hypothesis for each disorder before processing continues. If there is more than one hypothesis contributing to the diagnosis, they are ranked according to the degree of belief in each alternative at the 'diagnosis' level of the physiological diagnosis panel. The physiological diagnosis obtained from this process is transferred to the lowest level of the clinical diagnosis panel by the 'transfer data' knowledge source. This can be compared with the diagnosis entered by the clinician via the 'input diagnosis' knowledge source and written to the highest level of the clinical diagnosis panel. The knowledge source 'predict disorders' processes the expected set of disorders for each diagnosis entered by the clinician and passes them to the 'hypothesis' level of the panel. It is these hypotheses which are compared with the output from the physiological diagnosis panel. The 'critique diagnosis' knowledge source is responsible for passing the conclusions drawn by the comparison to the database for interrogation by the user.

9.12 Transcutaneous oxygen and carbon dioxide electrodes

Heated electrodes for the measurement on the skin as an approximation for the arterial oxygen or carbon dioxide tension are in widespread use for the continuous non-invasive monitoring of blood-gas tensions. Essentially, the operating principles of the electrodes are similar to those employed in the membrane-covered electrodes employed in conventional blood-gas analysers. However, the construction is compact to allow for each electrode to be attached to the skin by means of a double-sided adhesive ring. Each electrode housing also contains a low voltage heater and a thermistor temperature sensor allowing the electrode to be maintained at a constant preset temperature within the range 42 to 45 degrees Celsius.

With the transcutaneous electrodes heated, usually to 44 degrees Celsius, full vasodilation of the underlying capillary bed occurs and the resulting blood flow exceeds the local metabolic requirements of the tissue, allowing the transcutaneous gas tensions to approximate to the corresponding arterial values. The heating power supplied to the electrode assembly to maintain the preset temperature is related to the magnitude of the blood flow beneath the electrode. The heating power is continuously monitored and if this starts to decrease it indicates that a peripheral circulation shut-down is commencing. Under these conditions the transcutaneous blood-gas tensions will be unreliable.

Care must be taken not to exceed temperatures of 45 degrees Celsius in order to avoid burning the skin. Particular care is required with the delicate skin of neonates, and operation at 42 degrees Celsius may be desirable with the electrode site changed every few hours.

To prevent overheating, the heating power is disconnected and an error message displayed within 30 seconds indicating one of the following fault conditions: the temperature exceeeds 46 degrees Celsius; the temperature is out of range; the temperature sensor is broken or short-circuited; the microprocessor operation is interrupted. Alarms are also provided to indicate if the measured tensions are outside preset upper and lower limits with an 8-second delay before an alarm sounds to allow for nursing interventions.

The electrodes can be pre-calibrated by immersing them in a water bath at the electrode's operating temperature, bubbling air through the water and making the appropriate corrections in the partial pressure calculation for the barometric pressure and the presence of water vapour. The zero can be set by bubbling through with nitrogen. Alternatively, the transcutaneous electrodes can be calibrated against the tension values obtained from a sample of the patient's arterial blood and a conventional blood-gas analyser.

Transcutaneous oxygen electrodes are widely used with neonates following a difficult delivery, when respiratory problems occur or where the mother's condition during pregnancy may have adversely affected the fetus. The 95% response time for a transcutaneous oxygen electrode fitted with a 25 micrometre thick Teflon membrane would be typically 12 to 18 seconds.

Clearly, the transcutaneous values, considering all types of patient, will not be as accurate as the corresponding arterial values, but are valuable for monitoring trends. The transcutaneous electrodes should be sited over a region of well-perfused tissue, and they are often placed on the thorax. Combined transcutaneous oxygen and carbon dioxide electrodes have been developed and these are useful in the management of patients having automatic ventilation of the lungs. A typical range for a transcutaneous oxygen electrode would be 0 to 99.9 kPa (0 to 751 mm Hg) and for a transcutaneous carbon dioxide electrode 0 to 20 kPa (0 to 150 mm Hg).

9.13 The use of gastric intramucosal pH as a therapeutic index of tissue oxygenation in critically ill patients

Gutierrez et al. (Gutierrez, G., Palizas, F., Doglio, G., Wainstein, N., Gallesio, A., Pacin, J., Dubin, A., Schiavi E., Jorge, M., Pusajo, J., Klein, F., San Roman, E., Dorfman, B., Shottlender, J. and Giniger, R. (1992) 'Gastric intramucosal pH as a therapeutic index of tissue oxygenation in critically ill patients', The Lancet, 339, 195–9), state that falls in gastric intramucosal pH (pHi) are associated with morbidity and mortality in patients admitted to intensive care units. They confirmed that the outcome for such patients can be improved by means of therapy guided by changes in pHi and aimed at improving systemic oxygen availability.

The monitoring of pHi is undertaken by means of a tonometer having a unique identification number and placed in the patient's stomach. The tonometer consists of a saline-filled silicone rubber balloon attached to the distal end of a standard nasogastric tube. The silicone rubber balloon was filled with 2.5 ml of 0.9% saline. After sufficient time was allowed for equilibration to occur between the carbon dioxide tension of the saline and the gastric lumen, anaerobic samples of the tonometer saline and of arterial blood were taken simultaneously and analysed and pHi calculated using a modification of the Henderson-Hasselbach equation pHi = 6.1 + log10 (Arterial bicarbonate concentration (F) × tonometer saline PCO_2)) where F is a time-dependent factor for partly equilibrated samples and is provided by the manufacturer of the tonometer. pHi guided resuscitation did not prove successful for patients having a low pHi (below 7.35) on admission but for those with a normal pHi on admission (7.35 or higher) it may have helped to avoid splanchnic hypoxia and it may also have prevented the development of a systemic oxygen deficit. For those patients admitted with a low pHi for treatment to improve systemic oxygen availability there was a 37% survival rate which compared with 58% for treated patients admitted with a normal pHi.

9.14 Fuel cell and polarographic oxygen monitors

Anaesthetic machines are normally fitted with an oxygen analyser and these are also useful for checking on the oxygen concentration in the atmosphere of oxygen tents and incubators. More sophisticated anaesthetic gas-mixture monitors can also measure nitrous oxide, carbon dioxide and a volatile anaesthetic agent such as enflurane using techniques such as acoustic spectrometry or a combination of a paramagnetic oxygen analyser with an infra-red absorption system for the other components of the mixture. Compact oxygen monitors may be of the polarographic oxygen-electrode type, fitted with a membrane, but they are also likely to be of the fuel-cell type because of the relatively rugged construction. The cell consumes oxygen as fuel and generates an electric current which is proportional to the concentration of oxygen. A range of 0–100% oxygen can be obtained with an accuracy of plus or minus 2% of full scale or plus or minus 5% of the actual reading. A 90% response time of better than ten seconds and a lifetime of at least ten months in 100% oxygen are claimed. Both high and low oxygen-concentration alarms can be set, with the low alarm being automatically activated when the oxygen concentration falls below 18%.

It has to be remembered that the calibration of nearly all electrochemical gas sensors is pressure sensitive. The normal cyclic pressure occurring within a breathing system resulting from spontaneous respiration will not significantly affect the oxygen concentration reading of the sensor. However, it has been shown an oxygen sensor produced a reading which was high when the sensor was located between the common gas outlet of an anaesthetic machine and the inlet to a minute volume-divider type of ventilator when the inlet pressure was in the range 33–55 kilopascals. Thus, oxygen sensors in breathing systems should be located as near as possible to the patient and, if possible, downstream of all other items of equipment.

9.15 Catheter-tip oxygen sensors

Miniature Clark-type polarographic oxygen sensors mounted at the tip of a suitable catheter have been developed for use in the umbilical artery of neonates. Murphy, A. P. and Rolfe, P. (1992) 'Intravascular oxygen sensor with polyetherurethane membrane: in vitro performance', *Medical and Biological Engineering and Computing*, **30**, 121–2, describe such a device with a tip diameter of 0.9 mm with a polyetherurethane membrane which is said to be biocompatible, non-thrombogenic and permeable to oxygen.

9.16 Gas monitors for use with an extracorporeal circulation

Needle-type oxygen and carbon dioxide electrodes have been developed for insertion into the circuit of a heart-lung machine to enable continuous monitoring of the blood-gas tensions during open-heart surgery. An alternative approach comprises a probe which can be connected to the oxygenator by means of a fibre optic 1.5 metres in length linking with a digital display unit indicating the venous haemoglobin oxygen saturation percentage and the haematocrit. The system can operate over a blood-flow rate of 1 to 6 litres per minute and blood temperature of 15 to 37 degrees Celsius with a range of 40–95% oxygen saturation and 15–35% haematocrit. The venous saturation describes the accuracy of perfusion and the haematocrit provides information on the state of the patient's haemodilution.

9.17 Pulse oximeters

The percentage oxygen saturation of blood is defined as the percentage of haemoglobin which is in the form of oxyhaemoglobin. Oxygen can be reversibly bound to haemoglobin and the percentage of the haemoglobin which is saturated with oxygen is given by the ratio: (ml of oxygen actually carried per 100 ml of blood) $\times$ 100% / (ml of oxygen carried by haemoglobin per 100 ml of blood when fully saturated). The instrument used to measure percentage oxygen saturation is an oximeter. In the case of a laboratory type of oximeter the blood sample is contained in an optical cuvette which is transilluminated alternatively with two beams of light having wavelengths of 660 and 940 nanometres which are determined by means of optical filters. The ratio of the intensities of the transmitted light at these two wavelengths is proportional to the percentage oxygen saturation of the sample.

The availability of compact solid-state light-emitting diodes capable of generating a strong emission of infra-red light in approximately the wavelength regions required and of being rapidly pulsed on and off under microprocessor program-control has led to the rapid development of pulse oximeters which have opened up the prospects for oxygen saturation monitoring in intensive care situations. The light sources and infra-red detector can be mounted in a compact and lightweight finger or toe probe. These body sites are chosen because they are normally well-perfused. Light at the specific wavelengths emitted by the infra-red light-emitting diodes passes through the tissue and falls on to a photodetector. The output from the detector consists of a pulsatile (a.c.) component resulting from pulsations in the arterial perfusion superimposed upon a steady component (d.c.) due to the passage of light through non-pulsatile tissue and venous blood. The pulse oximeter functions by using the d.c. signal at each wavelength to normalize the corresponding a.c. signals. The ratio of the a.c. signals is then converted into an oxygen percentage saturation reading using an algorithm stored in the memory of the oximeter's microcomputer.

A typical pulse oximeter would have two 3-digit 7 segment light-emitting diode digital displays for 0–100% saturation and a pulse rate indication of 20 to 250 beats per minute. An LED display of the pulse amplitude is also available. An accuracy of plus or minus 2% saturation over the range 70–100% saturation is claimed.

A mains-power supply or a sealed lead-acid 12-volt battery can be selected. Preset alarms can be brought into play for high or low oxygen-saturation values and pulse rates. The choice of sensor available is likely to include adhesive, sterile and disposable types. There is also likely to be a facility to allow an optional printer to be connected. Pulse oximeters are very convenient devices for monitoring oxygen saturation values under intensive therapy circumstances with a real-time display of values. However, it must be remembered that the lack of an optical cuvette with its fixed geometry renders this type of oximeter inherently less accurate than a laboratory type of oximeter which requires in vitro blood samples.

Oximeters are calibrated to display the percentage saturation of functional haemoglobin, the normal values being 94–98%. Significant concentrations of dysfunctional haemoglobins such as methaemoglobin (normal concentrations 0.2 to 0.6%) and carboxy haemoglobin (normal concentrations for non-smokers 0–0.8%) can affect the accuracy. However, some versions of laboratory oximeters are designed to be able to measure the concentrations of both normal and dysfunctional haemoglobins. Dyes such as indocyanine green which has been used for cardiac-output determinations can also affect the accuracy of oximeters. Reynolds, K. J., Moyle, J. T. B., Gale, L. B., Sykes, M. K. and Hahn, C. E. W. (1992) 'In vitro performance test system for pulse oximeters', *Medical and Biological Engineering and Computing*, **30**, 629–35, have described a calibration system for use with pulse oximeters which is capable of use down to saturation values of less than 40%.

With some forms of pulse oximeter it is possible to synchronize the individual readings with each R-wave of the patient's electrocardiogram. This possibility can be helpful when the oximeter is having difficulty in synchronizing to the patient's peripheral pulse waveform. It is reassuring to observe that the patient has an adequate peripheral circulation enabling the oximeter to follow beat-by-beat saturation values. For the generation of trend plots, oximeters are available with data storage capable of holding saturation and pulse-rate values obtained at five-second intervals over a 12-hour period. Analogue and digital outputs are provided for interfacing to central station patient-monitoring systems, records and computers.

9.18 Applications of pulse oximeters

Pulse oximeters are widely encountered during anaesthesia, intensive therapy for patients suffering from respiratory insufficiency and in special care baby units where problems may arise with infants born with immature lungs or prone to the Sudden Infant Death Syndrome (SIDS).

Southall, D. P. and Samuels, M. (1992) 'Inappropriate sensor application in pulse oximetry', *The Lancet*, **340**, 481–2 describe a recording of what appeared to be a prolonged episode of hypoxaemia (80–82% saturation) in a sleeping ten-week-old infant, the oximeter appearing to produce good signals. The sensor was secured to a big toe by means of compliant tape. A close examination revealed that a proportion of the light emitted by the sensor was 'shunting' past the tissue bed directly on to the receiving photodiodes of the sensor. On readjustment of the position of the sensor on the big toe, oxygen-saturation values of 97–100% were obtained. Southall and Samuels point out that a discrepancy of this magnitude could lead to the excessive administration of inspired oxygen. In the pre-term infant there would be a risk of retinopathy and other possible manifestations of oxygen toxicity. Staff need to be well-trained in the use of pulse oximeters, and regular checks need to be made on the positioning of the sensor with fresh adhesive used to secure the sensor to the patient to avoid the possibility of slippage occurring after prolonged monitoring.

Poets, C. F., Seidenberg, J. and Von Der Hardt, H. (1993) 'Failure of pulse oximeter to detect sensor detachment', *The Lancet*, **341**, 44, found that a pulse oximeter was providing apparently normal oxygen saturation and pulse signals despite a complete detachment of the sensor from the skin of a six-week-old pre-term infant! It was noted that the sensor which had been attached to the infant's foot by means of a fixation wrap provided by the manufacturer, had come off and was lying face-up in the incubator 10 cm distant from the infant. The pulsatile signal being produced was at a rate almost identical with the infant's heart rate and the oxygen saturation values displayed were constantly 98–99%. On close inspection it was evident that the 'pulse' waveforms were quite different from that produced with patients. The pulsations disappeared immediately when the room lights were extinguished.

If an infant is not in an incubator, it is necessary to ensure that a finger or toe to which is attached a pulse-oximeter probe must not be allowed to become so cool that there is a marked reduction in the peripheral circulation which will affect the oximeter's reading.

9.19 Renal dialysis

9.19.1 Haemodialysis

Patients in renal failure or with severely reduced renal function suffer from the effects of increased concentrations of sodium, potassium, chloride and urea in their extracellular fluid. Substitutes for renal function are the use of haemodialysis in which an artificial kidney machine is employed to adjust the concentrations of peritoneal dialysis. In these patients blood pH and electrolyte determinations are important to ensure that the patient remains in a satisfactory condition throughout the therapy.

A 70 kg patient will contain some 40 litres of water and of this some 27 litres is contained within the cells as intracellular fluid (ICF) while some 13 litres is outside the cells in the extracellular fluid (ECF). Of this, most is located between the cells as the interstitial fluid while the remainder comprises body fluids such as blood (which contains some three litres of water), lymph, gastric juices and urine. The ICF serves as a reservoir of raw materials for sustaining metabolic processes. The ECF functions as a transport system for the body. In healthy tissues fuels for metabolism and the resulting waste products are transported to and fro from the cells via the ECF which maintains the correct composition of the ICF.

Important components of both the ICF and the ECF are electrolytes such as sodium and potassium. Significant disturbances of the patient's electrolyte concentrations can result in symptoms such as coma, convulsions, cramp, diarrhoea, heart failure and vomiting. The dominant positively charged ion in the ECF is sodium Na^+. Its concentration in a normal patient is regulated by the endocrine and renal systems under the control of the brain. For patients with an impaired or absent renal function, renal dialysis is employed to correct the electrolyte balance for the whole body by adjusting the concentration of ions in the small fraction of the body's fluid contained in the blood.

During dialysis the sodium ion concentration in the serum is adjusted to correspond with that of the dialysing fluid. This fluid is pumped past one side of the dialyser's semi-permeable membrane while the patient's blood is pumped past on the other side. The material chosen for the membrane is sufficiently porous to allow all the plasma constituents except the plasma proteins to diffuse freely in both directions.

In the case of diffusion the amount of a substance which transfers depends on a) the concentration gradient of that substance existing across the membrane; b) the molecular size since smaller molecules will diffuse more rapidly than larger molecules; and c) the length of time for which the fluids are in contact with the surface of the membrane. If the level of Na^+ in the ECF is higher than that of the dialysing fluid, sodium ions will diffuse through the membrane from the blood to the dialysing fluid. The ions removed from the serum are replaced from the ICF. If the rate of replacement is insufficient, the difference in the concentrations of Na^+ between the ICF and the serum can generate an osmotic pressure driving water from the blood into the tissues which leads to tissue oedema and to hypotension. In acetate dialysis the dialysing fluid is a sodium acetate buffer while in bicarbonate dialysis it is a sodium bicarbonate buffer. The dialysing fluid is an electrolyte solution which is usually made up as needed by diluting one or more concentrated solutions. Dialysing fluid is the term usually applied to fresh fluid, while dialysate covers fresh or used solution.

The dialyser section of the artificial kidney contains a semi-permeable membrane across which both diffusion and ultrafiltration of impurities and waste in the blood can occur. The dialyser section is usually in the form of a disposable (single use) coil. Renal dialysis can be accomplished by means of either a single-needle or a twin-needle technique. In the single-needle technique, blood is alternately taken from and returned to the patient via a single needle. The blood flow is controlled by a pair of peristaltic pumps or by a single pump plus a pair of automatic line clamps. In the case of the twin-needle technique, blood is continuously removed from and returned to the patient via two separate needles. The flow of blood to the dialyser can be controlled by a single peristaltic pump. Connection to the arterial circulation for input to the dialyser and to the venous circulation for return flow from the dialyser on a long-term basis can be accomplished via a surgically provided arterio-venous fistula at the wrist.

Ultrafiltration involves the transfer of fluid across the semi-permeable membrane as a result of a pressure gradient across the membrane. The required pressure gradient can be accomplished by pressurizing the fluid on one side of the membrane or depressurizing the fluid on the other side. In some haemodialysis systems it is possible to remove excess fluid from the patient as an option by ultrafiltration without the simultaneous diffusion of particles through the membrane. Fluid replacement, by means of a heated sterile electrolyte solution, can be used to substitute for the fluid lost by ultrafiltration. A fluid-balancing device may be used in conjunction with ultrafiltration. It monitors the mass of fluid removed from the patient and controls the delivery of the replacement (substitution fluid). The fluid-balancing system is shown in Figure 9.9 and will be described in more detail later in this section.

Water crossing the membrane during ultrafiltration can carry with it any solutes which are small enough to pass through the pores of the membrane. For ultrafiltration a highly permeable membrane is employed having an ultrafiltration coefficient of approximately 50 ml per hour per mmHg in contrast to the corresponding value of some 10 ml per hour per mmHg for a standard haemodialysis membrane.

Small and middle-sized molecules of molecular weights up to 40 000 can pass easily through the high permeability membrane. This process is known as convection or 'solvent drag'. Since diffusion is not required there is no need for the presence of dialysing fluid. Convection is the principal mechanism for the removal of waste products in the technique of haemofiltration. This combination of ultrafiltration, convection and fluid replacement may reduce many of the side-effects associated with haemodialysis, but the cost of the sterile replacement fluid required for the patient may be prohibitive. A combination of haemodialysis and haemofiltration is known as haemodiafiltration. Good accounts of suitable equipment for haemodialysis and ultrafiltration appear in Evaluation Reports 69 (August 1991) and 119 (March 1992) published by the Medical Devices Directorate of the UK's Department of Health in London.

The electrical conductivity of the dialysing fluid (usually expressed in units of milli-siemens per cm) is continuously monitored as a measure of

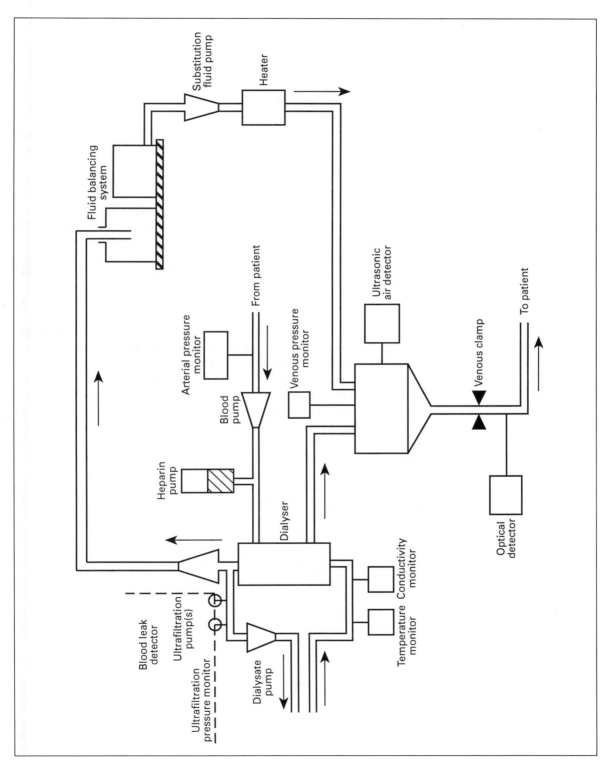

Figure 9.9 Simplified diagram of a Fresnius haemodialyser fitted with a fluid-balancing system.

the electrolyte concentration of the fluid. A separate heparin pump adds anti-coagulant to the patient's blood at a preset rate to prevent clotting at a rate of 0.5 to 10 ml per hour. Haemodialysers incorporate a number of protective systems to warn against: mains failure; water-supply failure; change of dialysate temperature outside a 3–4 degrees Celsius band around the preset value; conductivity of the dialysate outside preset limits; similarly for dialysate flow-rate, transmembrane pressure, arterial and venous pressures, blood-pump stoppage, leakage of blood into the dialysate, fluid-level drop or presence of bubbles/froth and heparin pump empty.

Some haemodialysers incorporate hot rinse and disinfection modes. Sodium hypochlorite or formalin can be used as disinfectants. Section 2.16 of British Standard 5724 adapts the Standard specifically for haemodialysis systems which fall within its scope. For a dialysing fluid flow rate of 300 ml per minute, typical clearances by haemodialysis might be: urea 175 ml per minute; creatinine 140 ml per minute; phosphate 116 ml per minute for single-and twin-needle modes of operation. A maximum ultrafiltration rate of 200 ml per minute is attainable.

Some types of haemodialyser provide a variable sodium facility in which the dialysing fluid has a high Na^+ concentration at the commencement of dialysis when the patient's serum concentration can also be high. This matches the removal of sodium from the serum to a rate which can be matched by replacement from the interstitial fluid. The concentration of Na^+ in the dialysing fluid is gradually reduced to leave the patient with an acceptable Na^+ concentration in the serum at the end of dialysis. Most sodium variation systems operate by simply altering the mixing ratio of dialysate concentrate to water. Increasing the concentration of sodium ions will thus also increase the concentrations of all the electrolyte present in the dialysate.

Figure 9.9 is a block diagram of a sophisticated haemodialysis system complete with fluid-balancing system. The arterial line to the blood pump has an arterial pressure monitor and a separate pump adds heparin to the blood. After passing by one side of the dialyser's membrane the blood returns to the venous line via a venous-pressure monitor, ultrasonic air-bubble detector, venous clamp and optical blood-level detector. The dialysate pump circulates heated, mixed and degassed dialysate around the other side of the membrane via temperature and conductivity monitors. If ultrafiltration is used, excess fluid accumulating via the dialyser's membrane is diverted to the reservoir of the fluid-balancing system and causes a corresponding amount of heated substitution fluid to be returned to the venous line.

9.19.2 Peritoneal dialysis

Haemodialysis systems for chronic use are normally located in a multi-system renal unit in a hospital, or for selected individual patients, at home. Patients are dialysed for periods of several hours two or three times per week. Peritoneal dialysis is suitable for short-term *ad hoc* use for patients with inadequate renal function during intensive care. The patient's peritoneal cavity is intermittently filled with dialysing fluid, and dialysis occurs across the natural membrane – the peritoneum. Peritoneal dialysis is not as efficient as a haemodialyser and is used for emergency therapy.

Pre-heated dialysing fluid is fed under gravity to and from the patient's peritoneal cavity. The transferred volume is determined by weighing the appropriate fluid-containing bag before and after the transfer phase of treatment. A pump is used to transfer fluid from the supply to the heater bag and from the drain bag to waste. It is possible to set the equipment to automatically cycle through a preset number of cycles of filling and emptying the peritoneal cavity. The fill time can be adjusted between 1 to 99 minutes, as can the drain time, with a dwell time for fluid in the peritoneal cavity of 0 to 590 minutes. For an adult, a volume of 2 litres might be transferred per cycle. Alarm facilities cover mains failure, dialysing fluid temperature and fluid overfill.

Figure 9.10 shows the block diagram of a Gambro PD 100 peritoneal dialysis equipment. It consists of a mobile stand on which are mounted the microprocessor control unit and the drain-valve assembly of the fluid cycler. The height of the control unit can be varied to provide the required gravitational head for fluid transfer. Up to 6 bags of dialysing fluid can be suspended from the top of the stand. Fluid flow is controlled by electro-mechanical pinch valves. The patient fill valve is opened to permit fluid from the heater bag to flow to the patient during the fill/dwell phase of the

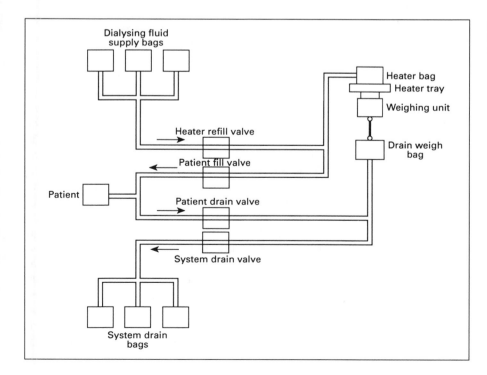

Figure 9.10 Block diagram of Gambro PD 100 peritoneal dialysis equipment.

fluid cycle. The quantity of fluid transferred to the patient is measured from the change in weight of the heater bag. When the patient fill is complete, the heater refill valve is opened, allowing the heater bag to be topped up from the suspended fluid bags. During the drain phase, the patient drain valve is opened, allowing fluid to drain from the patient into the drain bag which is also weighed. At the end of the drain phase the system drain valve opens, allowing the fluid in the drain bag to flow to waste. The heater tray maintains the heater bag at approximately 37 degrees Celsius. A good account of this system appears in Evaluation Report 80 (September 1991) published by the Medical Devices Directorate of the UK's Department of Health in London.

Both haemodialysis and peritoneal dialysis require a high degree of care in terms of setting-up the equipment, maintaining sterility during intensive use by a large number of patients and monitoring the patient's condition during what can be powerful therapy. This involves cooperation between the patient, medical and nursing staff, medical-physics staff (for equipment maintenance) and artificial kidney assistants, together with the services of the hospital's chemical-pathology department for the estimation of analytes such as urea and phosphate. The criteria to be considered when selecting haemodialysis systems include: compliance with the relevant safety standards; performance; reliability; servicing; user-friendliness; size; weight; noise output; range of facilities available; and initial purchase price and running costs.

9.20 The use of an extracorporeal membrane oxygenator (ECMO)

Diffusion of molecules across a semi-permeable membrane with the patient's blood flowing on one side of the membrane and dialysing fluid on the other is a feature of haemodialysis. In the normal lung gas exchange results from the diffusion of carbon dioxide and oxygen across the alveolar membrane to and from central venous blood and alveolar gas. It is possible, for emergency purposes, to replace the lungs with an extracorporeal membrane oxygenator.

Situations do arise where a marked deterioration develops in the gas-exchange properties of a patient's lungs leading to a life-threatening oxygen desaturation. If, with suitable therapy, the condition can be substantially reversed there arises a requirement for a mechanical oxygenator to take over the role of the lungs. A suitable device is a membrane type of oxygenator. Unlike the case of a full extracorporeal circulation as used in cardiac surgery, with the ECMO the patient's heart provides the circulation. Tebbatt, A., Pearson, G., Firmin, R. K. and Reeves, R. (1992) 'Paediatric ECMO – a case study', *The Perfusionist*, **16**, 19, describe the use of a membrane oxygenator with a 5.5-year-old child suffering from chicken pox pneumonia. In this form of therapy, the regular monitoring of the patient's blood-gases is important.

9.21 Extracorporeal cardio-pulmonary bypass

When it is required to deliberately stop the pumping action of the heart for an extended period, for example, to permit valve replacement, the correction of congenital abnormalities or a cardiac transplant, a combination of an oxygenator together with peristaltic pumps to take over the arterial and venous circulations is employed in the form of a so-called heart-lung machine. The oxygen consumption requirements of the patient's heart can be reduced by rendering the patient hypothermic by means of electric fans and swabbing the patient with chilled water or the use of a mattress fitted with tubes for the circulation of chilled water.

The bypass equipment is operated by skilled perfusionists, often led by a consultant anaesthetist. The heart is initially stopped from beating at the appropriate stage of the surgical procedure by passing a controlled amount of mains-frequency current through it and in due course restarted by using a defibrillator. During the procedure, careful monitoring of blood pressures, body temperature, the ECG and the EEG is necessary, together with blood-gas and electrolyte determinations.

10 Infusion pumps and controllers

10.1 Introduction

Patients in intensive care situations regularly require the administration of known volumes of drugs and fluids such as sodium or potassium chloride and crystalloid solutions by means of an intra-venous infusion which proceeds at a known predetermined rate and which is readily controllable.

The United Kingdom's Department of Health has defined four main categories for the use of infusion devices: neonatal infusions; high risk infusions; lower risk infusions and ambulatory infusions. Devices recommended for the administration of neonatal infusions could be used for all the other applications, providing that the flow-rate range available is adequate. Devices recommended for high risk infusions could also be used for lower risk infusions. However, on the contrary, devices designed to administer low risk infusions must not be used for neonatal or high risk infusions. Devices designed for use with ambulatory infusions are carried on the person and are battery or clockwork powered. Health Circular (Hazard) (91) 12, 5 July 1991 from the Medical Devices Directorate of the UK's Department of Health reports that the effect of dropping a clockwork syringe driver resulted in the death of the patient from an overdose of diamorphine over a 12-hour period. Furthermore, the device had not been regularly checked or maintained by the hospital.

Infusion devices are commonly encountered in intensive care situations and on wards so that medical, nursing and biomedical equipment staff all need to understand how they should be set up, the flow-rate correctly adjusted and checks made as necessary to ensure that the unit is performing as required. The Department of Health's Medical Devices Directorate makes the assumption that all neonatal infusions fall into the high risk category and that a smooth delivery and consistency of flow, the availability of low flow rates with the possibility of 0.1 ml per hour increments, a high degree of accuracy for both short-term and long-term, comprehensive alarm facilities with very short alarm delays, a very low value of bolus on release of an occlusion and an automatic transfer to battery operation with failure of the mains electricity supply are all essential. With the exception of the low flow-rate availability, similar requirements occur for infusions using high risk agents such as cardiac amines and cytotoxic drugs for chemotherapy.

In the case of infusions such as those of simple electrolytes, antibiotics and parenteral nutrition fluids it may not be required to deliver a given volume of liquid in a precise time. The consistency of flow and a smooth delivery are not so important and a less comprehensive set of alarms may be acceptable. For these situations the use of a less sophisticated device designed for the lower risk infusions will save money. The main categories of acceptable infusion devices are: syringe pumps; volumetric pumps and drip rate gravity controllers. The use of drip-rate controllers was confined to intensive therapy units and manufacturers have now given preference to syringe pumps and volumetric pumps.

10.2 Syringe pumps

Essentially syringe pumps consist of a syringe of known volumetric capacity whose plunger is driven forward at a preset rate, having a long-term accuracy of within plus or minus 5% by means of an electric motor whose rotational speed can be accurately controlled. Various syringes can be fitted depending on the model of the pump. In some cases only a syringe from the manufacturer of the pump can be employed, e.g. one 50 ml IVAC syringe to produce a volume flow-rate range of 0.1 to 99.9 ml per hour from an IVAC pump. A battery-powered pump for use with ambulatory patients might make use of one syringe for the volume flow-rate range of 1 ml to 10 ml per hour, while one model which is powered by clockwork will only hold a single 10 ml syringe to provide three preset volume flow-rates of 0.416, 0.833 or 1.67 ml per hour. They would not be used for patients in the intensive care unit but with patients who have returned to a ward but still require pain-relief therapy.

It is obviously important that the user checks the manufacturer's instructions to be certain of the type of syringe which should be fitted to any particular pump for a given infusion. The construction of a syringe pump needs to be robust to ensure a reliable motion of the syringe barrel with easily readable and understandable controls under intensive care conditions and with alarm facilities available. Possible conditions which call for an alarm can include: the selection of an infusion rate of zero; the removal of the syringe; the disengagement of the driving carriage; the syringe becoming nearly empty; the emptying of the syringe; battery low; battery discharged; occlusion of the outlet; infusion not started; incorrect functioning. Both audible and visible alarms in various combinations are activated depending on the problem which has been detected.

The larger types of pumps are mains powered and may also be provided with an internal rechargeable battery for use when the patient is being moved from one location to another. In some models the plunger of the syringe is driven by a rotating lead screw-and-nut assembly powered by an electric motor having a tachometer feedback for speed control. The tachometer is a rotating device which generates an output signal which is proportional to the speed of the servo motor. This signal is compared continuously with a reference signal which is proportional to the desired speed. Any difference detected between the two signals causes the motor speed to be increased or decreased as appropriate until it attains the desired speed. Alternatively, a digital stepper motor may be employed. Here the motor does not continuously rotate but moves in a series of small steps driven by a train of digital pulses whose repetition rate can be altered to adjust the speed of rotation. The pump housing should be designed to be resistant to the ingress of spilled liquids and may be intended to mount on a flat horizontal surface or either vertically or horizontally on a pole used for supporting infusion fluid bags or bottles.

In the United Kingdom syringe pumps should conform in terms of electrical safety and the magnitude of leakage currents to the requirements of British Standard 5732: Part One (1974). The Medical Devices Bureau of the Department of Health has accepted that the provision of a mains switch is not essential for infusion pumps. Syringe pumps are particularly suited to the accurate infusion of fluids at low volume-flow rates. However, users of these pumps must ensure that the backlash of the plunger-drive mechanism has been fully taken up before the infusion is commenced. Otherwise there will be long delays before the flow to the patient begins, leading to the possibility of the vein chosen becoming occluded. In the case of one model of syringe pump set up to deliver one millilitre per hour, failure to take up the backlash resulted in a wait of 40 minutes for the flow-rate to attain 1 ml per hour.

If the pump manufacturer suggests in the operating instructions that the pump should be set to deliver a high volume flow rate for a short period prior to commencing the infusion in order to take up any backlash, it is essential that the user remembers to reset the pump to deliver at the required infusion rate before connection is made to the patient's vein, otherwise a gross over-infusion will occur. Alternatively, many infusion pumps are now fitted with a purge button which facilitates the taking up of any backlash. With some models, when the syringe is found to be almost empty the pump changes over to a low keep vein open (KVO) rate in order to maintain the vein in a condition of patency.

Syringe pumps which have a high occlusion alarm-pressure setting and are delivering a small volume flow rate will take a long time to indicate an occlusion alarm, e.g. 40 minutes to indicate an occlusion at a volume flow rate of 1 ml per hour. Syringe pumps capable of driving separately two syringes are more complicated in construction, but do allow the use of a 'piggy-back' technique in which a second infusion fluid is added to the primary fluid – normally by means of a Y-connector or manifold in the patient's line. Figure 10.1 illustrates the Graseby Medical Model 3100 syringe pump which is mains powered but also has a sealed lead-acid battery which can operate the pump for more than three hours. The flow rate is 0.1 to 199.9 ml per hour adjustable in 0.1 ml increments. In terms of British Standard 5724 Part One for electrical safety the syringe pump is

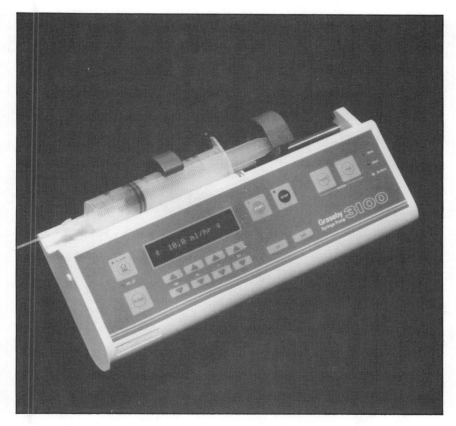

Figure 10.1 Graseby Medical
Model 3100 Syringe Pump.
(Courtesy Graseby Medical Ltd.)

Class II Type CF and is drip-proof. The accuracy of the syringe drive rate is plus or minus 2%.

10.3 Volumetric pumps

Volumetric pumps use a pumping arrangement such as a peristaltic finger or roller mechanism or a pair of pistons and cylinders driven at a known and controllable speed to provide a flow-rate accuracy of plus or minus 2%. Figure 10.2 illustrates the Graseby Medical Model 270/275 volumetric pump which is mains powered but also has a sealed lead-acid battery capable of powering the pump for 8 hours. The Model 270 version has a volume rate range of 1 to 999 ml per hour and the Model 271 is capable of 0.1 to 99.9 ml per hour. In terms of British Standard 5724 Part One these pumps are classified as Class II Type BF.

10.4 Drip-rate controllers

Drip-rate controllers are suitable for the majority of lower risk infusions which do not require volumetric accuracy. Some models can be used to

Figure 10.2 Graseby Medical Model 270/275 Volumetric Pump. (Courtesy Graseby Medical Ltd.)

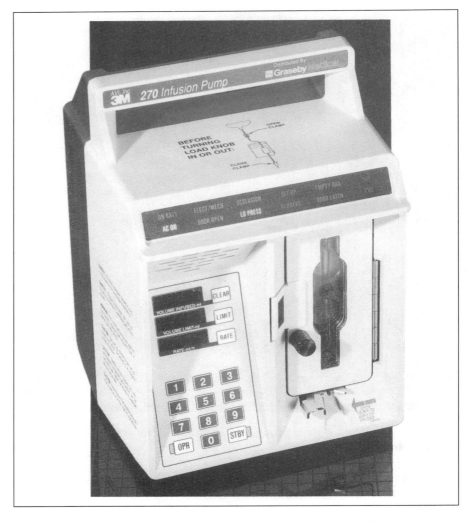

administer chemotherapy agents because of their particularly smooth and consistent delivery. The Department of Health makes the point that, contrary to accepted opinion, the infusion of parenteral nutrition fluids does not always require the application of pressures in excess of those available with gravity, and drip-rate controllers can be considered for this application. The better versions of drip-rate controller are sufficiently reliable that they can be entrusted with applications such as the infusion of 250 ml of a chemotherapy agent over a period of 30 minutes.

The main advantage cited for the use of gravity drip-rate controllers is that an early warning is provided of problems which arise at the site of the infusion. Modern versions of controller include a flow-status arrangement which warns of impending problems at the site of the infusion in advance of the final audible alarm. The system ignores any sudden and temporary increase occurring in the resistance to fluid flow and it is important that the attendant checks the site of the infusion when a warning is given.

There must be an adequate head of fluid in the supply line to the device for the flow rate required, typically a vertical height above the floor of 90 cm. A standard administration set provides a volume flow-rate of 20 drops per minute per ml of solutions such as simple electrolytes, normal saline and dextrose solutions up to 20% concentration. In use, the required drip rate is entered into the controller which is fitted with an infra-red or visible light-drop sensor. In one version, the associated flow controller incorporates a quiet-running d.c. motor which, via a gearbox, drives a pinch mechanism. This in turn controls the size of an orifice and thus the volume flow rate by compressing the tubing of the administration set. The desired drip rate is achieved within one or two minutes of the start-up, depending on the particular drip rate. Drip-rate controllers are suitable for the majority of low risk infusions which do not warrant volumetric accuracy. Modern versions are controlled by a microprocessor and are powered from the mains supply with an internal rechargeable battery back-up for use should the mains supply fail or if the patient is being moved.

10.5 Volumetric controllers

Volumetric controllers may be suitable for use with applications in adult intensive therapy units, renal dialysis units and general ward use where volume flow rates exceeding 5 ml per hour are required and where drug-potency considerations dictate a volumetric accuracy of plus or minus 5% over periods exceeding five minutes. For neonatal and high risk solutions with volume flow rates of less than 5 ml per hour the use of a syringe pump is preferred. Manufacturers are now giving preference to syringe pumps and volumetric pumps.

10.6 Enteral feeding pumps

Pumps for the provision of continuous enteral feeding are available based on various pumping mechanisms such as a rotary peristaltic mechanism or cassette/bellows. Mains supply is available, plus a battery back-up. Provision is made for pole-mounting or table-top operation. Alarms are available to cover eventualities such as occlusion of the feeding set, emptying of the feed bag, attempted rate of change of feeding and a low battery. A d.c. stepper motor is used to drive the peristaltic pump, with watchdog circuitry to monitor the motor-supply voltage and check for any condition which might cause runaway. The flow rate available might be 5 to 300 ml per hour adjustable in 5 ml per hour increments.

10.7 Implantable pumps

A new development is that of implantable pumps for applications such as the infusion of morphine sulphate for the treatment of intractable pain associated with cancer or the use of chemotherapy agents. One American design of implantable pump is approximately 70 mm in diameter by 25 mm in thickness. The complete system includes a small diameter catheter and a portable programmer. For the relief of chronic pain, morphine placed in a reservoir within the pump is delivered as programmed to the epidural space adjacent to the spinal cord via the catheter leading from the pump. After the pump has been surgically implanted under the skin of the patient's abdomen it can be programmed externally via a radiofrequency link to the programmer unit to deliver a daily dose of the drug. Normally, the pump's reservoir is refilled every two to six weeks by injection via a hypodermic needle through the skin into a self-sealing septum in the pump.

The complete arrangement comprises an 18 ml reservoir for the drug chosen, a miniature peristaltic pump, a microprocessor, a radiofrequency transmitter and output-coupling coil, an implanted receiver and coupling coil and a lithium battery as a power source for the implanted components which weigh approximately 180 grammes. The implanted components are hermetically sealed to prevent the ingress of body fluids and covered in silicone rubber to prevent rejection of the device by the patient as a foreign body. Figure 10.3 shows the Medtronic Synchromed implantable pump.

Figure 10.3 Synchromed Implantable Pump. (Courtesy Medtronic Inc.)

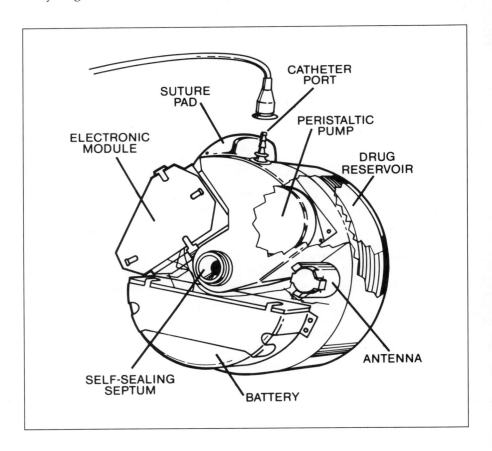

One application of the device is the intrathecal administration of drugs to the spinal cord to control severe spasticity of spinal cord origin in patients with injury of the spinal cord. After implantation under the skin in the abdominal area, the injection rate can be programmed externally via a radio link and the pump reservoir refilled at one-to-three-month intervals by needle injection.

10.8 The impact of European Communities legislation

From the commencement on 1 January 1993 of the European Single Market, under the European Communities Active Medical Devices Directive, most powered implantable medical devices (such as infusion pumps, cardiac pacemakers, stimulators, cochlea implants and artificial hearts) sold in the United Kingdom, including imports, must safeguard the clinical condition and safety of patients; not represent any risk to others; meet safety and efficacy requirements in their design, construction and materials used; have been designed and manufactured subject to independent checks; carry a 'CE mark' and provide instructions for use. As the new European Communities legislation covering medical devices takes effect, we can expect to see more and more devices approved in an EC country bearing the European Communities CE mark indicating their conformity with the Directive's 'essential requirements'. EC-recognized Test Houses carry out the assessments of conformity but it is the manufacturers who affix the CE mark and take legal responsibility for its use.

A second text on medical devices is proceeding through the European Communities decision-making process and is likely to apply from 1 July 1994. It will group products under four categories: Class I products which confer practically no risk to patient or attendant safety and do not need to be assessed by a Test House since manufacturers will self-certify; Class IIA and IIB devices which require assessment whose requirements are tougher as the product rises up the scale of risk; and Class III devices where failure could cause serious injury or death. Failures of Category III devices would have to be reported to national authorities which could pass details on to Brussels and other member states if Europe-wide product withdrawal became necessary. For National Health Service staff in the United Kingdom, the UK's Department of Health Medical Devices Directorate operates an incident-reporting service and associated Safety Action Bulletin. Hospitals encountering malfunction of a medical device are encouraged to report the details to the Directorate who may decide to initiate national warning procedures.

10.9 Computer-controlled infusions

For patients in an intensive care unit it is often important to maintain key physiological variables within predetermined limits. Blood pressure represents a good example. Sheppard, L. C. (1980) 'Computer control of the infusion of vaso-active drugs', *Annals of Biomedical Engineering*, **8**, 431, describes a closed-loop control system for use with cardiac patients who have become hypertensive following surgery. The infusion rate of sodium nitroprusside is automatically increased if the continuously measured arterial blood pressure exceeds a preset value. Once the blood pressure has decreased to a value considered by the clinical staff as 'normal' for that patient at that time, an appropriate decrease according to a set of rules is made in the rate of infusion of the hypotensive agent. Sheppard demonstrated that this approach can have a beneficial effect on patient care. In comparison with manual control of the infusion rate, the automatic system produced a closer control of the blood pressure and less hypotensive agent had to be administered. As a result the risk of complications arising from a hypertensive episode was reduced.

Similar approaches have been adopted to control the depth of anaesthesia using volatile anaesthetic agents. A computer-controlled fuel injector meters known amounts of the liquid agent into the measurement inspiratory flow of gas to the patient. The concentrations of anaesthetic agent are monitored by an infra-red sensor whose output feeds back to the controlling computer.

Incubators and infant radiant warmers

11

11.1 Introduction

Babies are prone to heat loss and the preservation of a suitable atmospheric environment to minimize cooling and maintain body temperature for extended periods is important. In addition to the maintenance of normothermia, nursing observation of the infant and ready access to it for therapeutic and cleansing purposes is essential. It may be necessary to provide monitoring of the oxygen concentration within the incubator in view of the possible hazards of retrolental fibroplasia. Phototherapy for jaundice may be required and facilities for automatic ventilation of the infant's lungs. The atmosphere within the incubator may need humidification if the baby is to stay in the incubator for some time.

Quite apart from the larger type of incubator which is normally resident in a special care baby unit (SCBU), it may be necessary to have available transport incubators designed to be suitable for deployment in ambulances or aircraft when infants at risk have to be transported back to a hospital for treatment which may include surgery. When short-term resuscitation involving vigorous procedures is required, it is impracticable to work on the infant while it is in an incubator. To permit unrestricted access to the naked baby, while still maintaining its body temperature, an infant radiant warmer unit is employed in which a servo-controlled infra-red heater warms the baby from above.

11.2 Conventional incubators

The aim of incubator designers is to provide a protective environment for the small babies using them which introduces minimal stress to their delicate thermoregulatory system. The energy input which has to be delivered to maintain their body temperature should be as low as possible. In comparison with full-term infants, premature babies have a body-surface area which is signficiantly greater in proportion to their body mass. They also have a smaller heat production but a greater heat loss. Thus, the function of the incubator is to compensate for these disadvantages.

Figure 11.1 Air-flow in a
double-walled infant ventilator.
(Courtesy Draeger Ltd.)

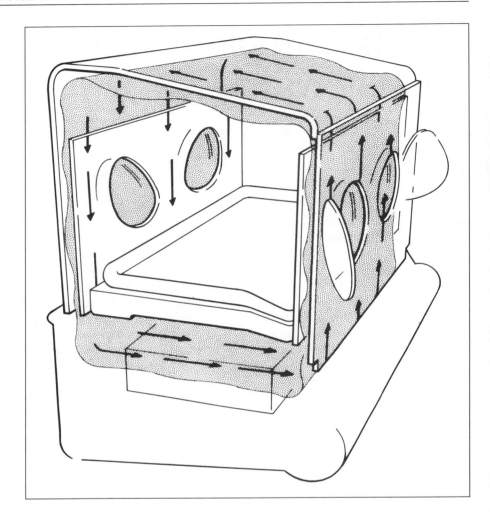

11.2.1 Incubator construction

Double clear plastic walls minimize heat losses from the baby by conduction, convection and radiation, and form part of the air-circulation system. Air is circulated continuously beneath the cot bed and between the pairs of walls, Figure 11.1. The roof of the incubator may be sloped in order to prevent reflections from ceiling lights from falling vertically on to the baby. Each long side of the incubator is fitted with two port doors and each short side with one port door to allow nursing access to the baby.

The cot bed can be adjusted from outside the incubator and can be inclined in either the head-up or the head-down position. The construction of the bed allows for the incorporation of an electronic weighing scale. The height of the incubator above the floor can be adjusted to suit individual attendants or to allow attendants to work with the baby while sitting, Figure 11.2. The incubator trolley should be mounted on a set of strong, large diameter castors fitted with brakes, to facilitate movement.

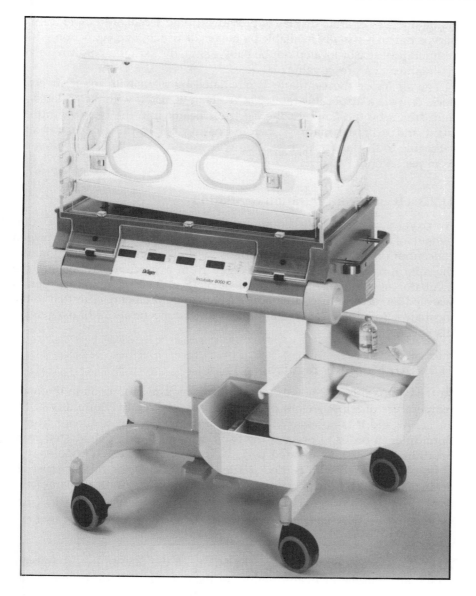

Figure 11.2 A modern infant incubator. (Courtesy Draeger Ltd.)

11.2.2 Temperature regulation

For a double-walled type of incubator fitted with a 400 watt heater, the warm-up time from an ambient temperature of 20 degrees Celsius to an operating temperature of 30 degrees Celsius is typically 35 minutes. The air temperature inside the incubator can be adjusted to be in the range 28 to 39 degrees Celsius. The opening of two of the hand ports to allow access to the baby should not lower the air temperature by more than 1 degree Celsius. In addition to a display of the temperature which is to be maintained, a separate display is provided of the actual air temperature. A servo control is usually available by means of which, in conjunction with a temperature sensor located on the baby's skin, the skin temperature can be maintained at a preset value.

The air inside the ventilator is circulated by a fan with room air being sucked in via a disposable filter. The fresh air is mixed with recirculated air and driven by the fan over the electrical heater into the baby's compartment and over the mattress, before passing below the baby's tray and returning to the fan for recirculation with an air velocity of approximately 8 cm per second.

11.2.3 Oxygen concentration regulation

An oxygen sensor with a liquid-crystal display may be used as a component of a modern incubator to both control and display the oxygen concentration of the incubator's atmosphere. A microprocessor monitors the appropriate volume flow of oxygen from a pipeline supply into the incubator to attain the preset level of oxygen. The incoming oxygen is warmed by passing through a heat exchanger before being admitted to the incubator. Both the measured and the desired concentrations of oxygen are displayed.

11.2.4 Air humidity regulation

At the comparatively high air temperatures required to maintain the body temperature of a low weight premature baby, the relative humidity of the air is low and it is necessary to add more water vapour to the air from a humidifier in order to prevent the baby from becoming dehydrated from breathing dry air for extended periods. In practice, a heated bubbler type of humidifier is fed with bottled sterile water and a water vapour sensor is arranged to control the percentage relative humidity at a preset value.

11.3 Alarms

Alarms are provided to monitor the failure of the fan, an excess ambient temperature in the incubator, failure of the temperature sensor and faulty electrical operation of the temperature-control system. Both audible and visual alarms may be provided in each case with the facility being available for muting the audible alarms. An alarm will also sound in the case of a failure of the mains power supply.

11.4 Accessories

Optional accessories for use with a sophisticated incubator will include items such as a head box for administering oxygen to the baby, a shelf and an infusion stand.

11.5 Electrical safety requirements for incubators

Incubators for use in the United Kingdom should satisfy the requirements applying to Type B equipment as specified in British Standard 5724 with those of Part One (1979) applying to all types and those of Section 2.21 (1983) applying to transport incubators.

11.6 Transport incubators

Transport incubators are designed to sustain the baby's environment while it is being transported back, usually by road or air, to a neonatal intensive care unit for resuscitation or to a suitable centre, perhaps for cardiac surgery, organ transplantation or neurological investigations. Transport incubators may also be used at peak periods in a special care baby unit to supplement the supply of conventional incubators. Hence, they are required to be capable of functioning from a mains electricity supply as well as an internal 12 volt sealed lead-acid battery or the 12 volt d.c. supply of an ambulance or aircraft.

The construction is relatively light weight, having a double-walled baby's compartment fitted with a transparent hinged acrylic canopy; a fan heater and temperature and oxygen controls; an observation lamp; an

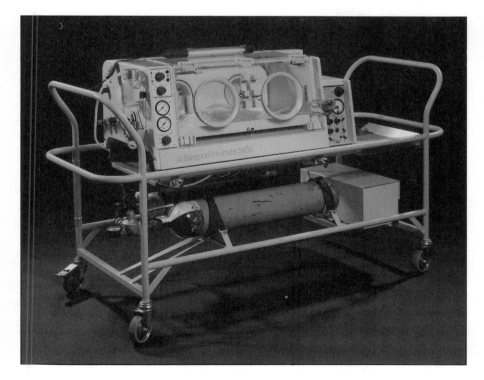

Figure 11.3 A transport incubator. (Courtesy Draeger Ltd.)

infusion stand; an oxygen-pressure regulator; a battery pack (sealed 12 volt with gel electrolyte) and a battery charger all mounted on a folding trolley, Figure 11.3. There may also be an air compressor and an automatic lung ventilator. Humidification can be provided from a small reservoir fitted with a sponge and containing sterile water. Some models of transport incubator are designed so that they can fit into an ambulance in place of a standard stretcher trolley and can easily be secured in place.

11.7 Infant radiant warmers

Infant radiant warmers are used when full access to the baby is required while vigorous resuscitation procedures are undertaken. A typical infant radiant warmer consists of a tilting bassinet above which is located an infra-red radiant heater which might consist of four ceramic panel heaters with a total power available of 600 watts. The maximum output power density is approximately 450 watts per square metre. The heater module includes an examination lamp, Figure 11.4. Since the maximum heater

Figure 11.4 Infant radiant warmer. (Courtesy Draeger Ltd.)

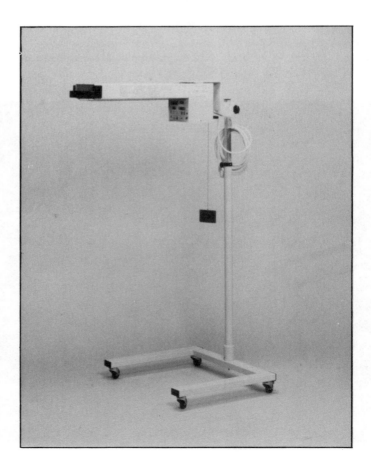

power exceeds 300 watts (which corresponds with a radiant heat emission of more than 10 milliwatts per square centimetre on the resting surface for the baby) a monitor with a visual and an audible alarm facility is automatically activated every 15 minutes to check the temperature of the baby and reset the heater if necessary. These items are mounted on a trolley with a drawer unit positioned below the bassinet. A shelf below the mattress can hold an X-ray film cassette.

The radiant warmer can be operated in either a manual or a servo-controlled mode where a skin sensor enables the baby's skin temperature to be maintained at a preset value, typically from 35 to 37.5 degrees Celsius in steps of 0.1 degrees Celsius with separate displays of the actual and preset temperatures. In the manual mode, the operator can adjust the power from zero to maximum in steps of 5%. The heater then operates for a period of 12 minutes when an audible alarm sounds. If no action is taken by the operator, heating continues for a further 3 minutes when the heater is automatically switched off and a further alarm is activated. Other alarms cover: mains power failure; electrical malfunction; deactivation of the heater during X-ray procedures; excessively high or low skin temperatures and failure of the temperature sensor when the warmer is operating in the servo mode. In some models a shelf may be provided to hold an infant-type ventilator, and provision may be made for mounting an oxygen cylinder, regulator and flowmeter to supply devices such as a resuscitator.

12 Defibrillators, external cardiac pacemakers and cardiac balloon pumps

12.1 Ventricular and atrial fibrillation

When the ventricles of a patient's heart fibrillate, the rhythmical coordinated contraction of the heart muscle associated with a recognizable ECG tracing ceases and the ECG degenerates to an entirely random tracing. A condition then exists of unsynchronized contractions of groups of individual cardiac muscle cells. Visually, the heart muscle appears to be 'squirming' rather than contracting in a regular fashion. The cessation of the pumping action causes the circulation of blood around the body to stop and death by anoxia occurs rapidly (irreversible brain damage occurs within a few minutes at normal body temperature) unless prompt corrective action is taken (as when electric shocks are applied, Figure 12.1) to restore a normal sinus rhythm.

Approximately 85% of cardiac arrest patients are in ventricular fibrillation for several minutes following collapse, unless they are already connected to an ECG monitor and the alarm facility draws the attention of trained attendants to the patient's condition. For each minute of fibrillation which elapses there is a decline of 7% to 10% in the probability that the patient will survive, with or without defibrillation. If defibrillation is delayed longer than 10 to 12 minutes, there is almost no chance of survival. This has led to the development of simplified and automated external defibrillators (AED) for minimally trained emergency personnel to deliver on-the-spot early defibrillation to patients in cardiac arrest: Cummins, R. O. (1989) 'From concept to standard-of-care? Review of the clinical experience with automated external defibrillators', *Annals of Emergency Medicine*, **18**, 1269–75.

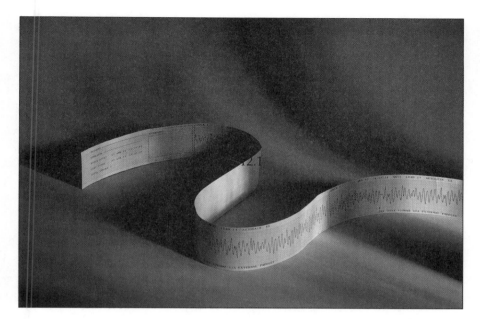

Figure 12.1 Output from a Hewett Packard Defibribrillator monitor showing 3 shocks for ventricular defibrillation administerd in less than 30 seconds. (By courtesy of Hewlett Packard Ltd.)

It is possible for the atria alone to fibrillate while the ventricles carry on beating synchronously to pump blood around the body. This is an undesirable state of affairs which may in time lead to ventricular fibrillation. Atrial fibrillation should be corrected as a planned procedure, whereas ventricular fibrillation is normally an emergency procedure unless it has been deliberately induced in cardiac surgery. The application of a suitable electrical countershock to the heart, either directly via electrodes touching the heart, or through the chest wall, can often reverse fibrillation into sinus rhythm and it can also restart a heart in asystole. These are both life-threatening conditions and the resuscitation equipment – which includes a defibrillator – must always be kept in good working order and available to be rushed to the patient wherever he or she may have collapsed in the hospital.

12.2 Operating principles of defibrillators

The shock to defibrillate the heart is supplied from a preset amount of electrical energy stored in a high voltage capacitor. The defibrillator is first 'armed' by the operator choosing the desired energy level and charging up the capacitor to this level from a high voltage supply built into the defibrillator. When it is time to defibrillate the patient, the pressing of the appropriate switch directs the chosen amount of energy to a pair of 'paddle' electrodes placed either on the chest wall or to spoon-shaped electrodes placed directly on the heart when the chest is open in cardiac surgery.

For an adult the shock required for ventricular defibrillation with paddle electrodes is usually of the order of 200 joules or more. For atrial defibrillation a smaller energy is used. In this case the discharge of the defibrillator is automatically synchronized to the R-wave of the patient's ECG via a delay so that the defibrillator fires before the appearance of the T-wave. This technique is known as cardioversion. Low energy cardioversion is also used to terminate haemodynamically unstable ventricular tachycardia.

12.3 The concept of stored and delivered energy

The unit of electrical energy is the joule and the energy expressed in joules stored in a capacitor of capacity C farads charged to V volts is equal to 0.5 × C × (V squared). Quite high voltages will appear on the capacitor at the higher energies. In the case of a 16 microfarad capacitor this must be charged to 1.5 kV to store 18 joules, to 2 kV for 32 joules, to 5 kV for 200 joules and to 7 kV for 392 joules. It is important that the capacitor is automatically discharged through a resistor after a preset time, if the defibrillator has not been fired, to avoid accidental shock to the operator if the electrodes are handled. This is necessary as a polycarbonate dielectric low leakage type of capacitor is used which will hold its charge for some time unless deliberately discharged. Similarly, it is usual to employ a spring-loaded push-button switch (or a pair of push-buttons) as part of the paddle electrodes, in order that the defibrillator cannot be fired unless the electrodes are making firm contact with the patient's skin, in order to minimize the possibility of burns to the skin.

In a capacitor discharge type of defibrillator, the capacitor is first arranged to be connected via the contacts of a sealed high voltage relay to the high voltage supply in order to 'arm' the defibrillator. When charging has been completed, actuating a push switch to 'fire' the defibrillator

Figure 12.2 Typical discharge waveform of 200 joules energy from a capacitor discharge defibrillator.

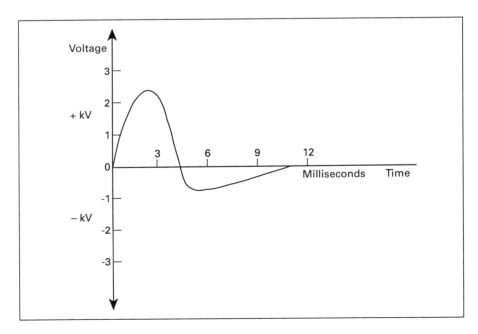

allows the relay to changeover and dump the charge stored on the capacitor (via an inductor) across the two patient electrodes. The action of the inductor (an iron cored coil) placed in series with the patient is to shape the pulse waveform used to defibrillate. As an example, a 40 microfarad capacitor charged to 5000 volts holds 500 joules of stored electrical energy. When the capacitor is discharged into a patient load of typically 50 ohms via a 0.1 Henry inductor, having a winding resistance of 50 ohms, only 250 joules is actually delivered to the patient. The remaining 250 joules are dissipated as heat in the resistance of the inductor's winding. The peak current which flows during the discharge is about 60 amperes and the peak voltage of the pulse generated is in excess of 2000 volts. Thus defibrillators need to be handled with respect. Figure 12.2 shows a typical discharge waveform.

A defibrillator is provided with an analogue meter or digital display of the delivered energy which will be available at the particular setting. The energy to be delivered can be preset by the operator using the meter or digital display. Depressing the charge button provides an immediate feedback to the user, in some models in terms of an audible click and a charging tone. When the preset energy level has been attained an audible tone sounds continuously and an indicator light flashes. If the defibrillator is not fired within a definite period, typically 20 seconds, the capacitor is automatically discharged via a dummy load.

12.4 Defibrillator electrodes

External (paddle-shaped) electrodes placed on the thorax so that the current flow passes through the heart are employed when the patient's chest is intact. In some models of defibrillator the paddle electrodes are spring loaded in such a way that the discharge of the defibrillator can only occur when the electrodes are pressed firmly on to the patient, thus reducing the possibility of causing localized skin burns.

Paddle electrodes are normally used in conjunction with electrically conducting electrode gel in order to minimize the risk of burns to the patient's skin. Pads of a porous non-woven fabric impregnated with conductive gel are commercially available in two sizes: 11.4 cm $\times$ 11.4 cm and 11.4 cm $\times$ 15.2 cm. The pads are first placed as required on the thorax and the paddle electrodes pressed down on to them. This saves the time involved in spreading gel on to the skin and leaves behind no slippery gel which might interfere with cardiopulmonary resuscitation efforts (CPR). With conventional paddle electrodes it is important not to spread the electrode gel too wide or the defibrillator charge may take a short-circuit path via the gel. Some models of defibrillator provide an indication of the contact resistance made by the electrodes with the patient. The operator fires the defibrillator by depressing a finger-operated switch mounted on the housing of one of the electrodes. In some models it is necessary to operate simultaneously a pair of push-button switches, one located on each paddle.

For use with the hearts of children, smaller paediatric paddle electrodes are employed. In some models the adult paddles can be twisted off to reveal the paediatric paddles. When the chest is open and the heart exposed, the heart is placed between a pair of metal spoon-shaped electrodes – each mounted on an insulated handle. A substantially smaller energy is required to defibrillate the heart when the electrodes touch the heart. It is arranged that these spoon electrodes can only plug into different sockets on the defibrillator from those used for the external paddle electrodes. The action of plugging them in automatically reduces the energy which can be delivered by the defibrillator in order to prevent burns to the heart.

12.5 Safety precautions when using defibrillators

The high voltage discharge produced by a defibrillator requires a high standard of insulation to protect the operator from a shock, and this means regular checking of the condition of both cables and electrodes. Defibrillator tests must also be regularly employed for checking that the delivered energy is as set by the operator. Defibrillators powered from sealed rechargeable batteries should be left permanently on trickle charge, ready for use. The battery pack is provided with protection against excess currents on both its input and output.

The battery must not be allowed to run down excessively if the defibrillator is to be used away from a mains supply since regular deep discharges and subsequent recharges may shorten the life of the battery. A protection circuit is provided to prevent the possibility of a deep discharge. If the mains supply is interrupted or disconnected the defibrillator will changeover automatically to battery power after a few seconds. Under rushed conditions there may not be time to remove electrodes and transducers from the patient before the defibrillator is fired. Such devices must be designed to withstand the defibrillator discharge or they may be permanently damaged.

12.6 The use of a cardioscope and ECG writer with a defibrillator

The achievement of defibrillation of the ventricles will be shown by the return of a coordinated pumping action and the presence of the associated ECG. Many defibrillators are provided with a built-in cathode ray tube display (cardioscope) of the ECG and a socket is usually provided to enable an ECG recorder to be plugged in. The bandwidth of the display is deliberately limited to about 0.25 to 25 Hz and the display can be frozen, on command, for 10 seconds for the inspection of details. A diagnostic ECG is best obtained via ECG electrodes on the thorax, but an indication of the ECG can be obtained by using the defibrillator's paddle electrodes to detect the ECG. Should the ECG cable not be connected, the source of the ECG should default to the paddle electrodes.

12.7 The technique of cardioversion

The more sophisticated models of defibrillator have a built-in cardioscope and synchronizer circuit to synchronize the discharge with the patient's ECG such that it occurs a definite time (typically 25 milliseconds) after the detection of an R-wave in the ECG. In the synchronized mode a lamp is arranged to flash for each R-wave detected. The monitor display is provided with a marker pulse to indicate at which point in the cardiac cycle the discharge would occur.

This form of synchronized discharge is known as cardioversion. It is used for atrial rather than ventricular fibrillation (where there is no ECG). A smaller energy, perhaps 25 J, is used than would be the case with ventricular fibrillation. The heart is vulnerable to ventricular fibrillation during the period of the T-wave of the ECG so that in cardioversion the defibrillator is always fired prior to the onset of the T-wave. Figure 12.3 shows a typical synchronized defibrillator-monitor.

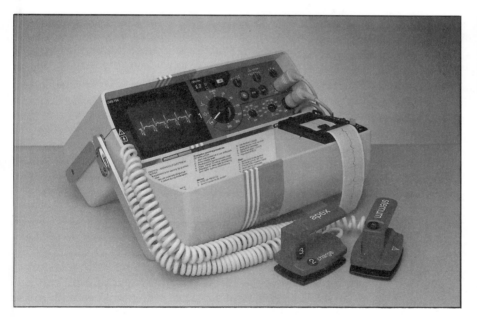

Figure 12.3 Simonsen & Weel Model DMS 700 Portable Synchronised Defibrillator-Monitor, maximum delivered energy 360 joules into a 50 ohm load. (Courtesy Simonsen & Weel.)

12.8 Electrode positions for defibrillation

For ventricular defibrillation the two paddle electrodes may be placed on the skin of the thorax in an anterio-posterior placement with the heart located between the electrodes. This may be inconvenient during resuscitation of the patient when an anterior-anterior placement is more suitable (one paddle to the right of the sternum at the second rib with the other at the xiphoid level at the mid-axillary line). Figure 12.4 shows a pair of paddle electrodes being applied to a pair of gel impregnated fabric pads.

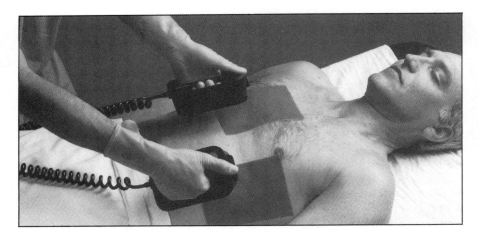

Figure 12.4 The anterior-anterior placement of defibrillator paddle electrodes in conjunction with fabric pads impregnated with electrode gel. (Courtesy of 3M Health Care.)

12.9 Power supplies

These can be normal mains supplies with provision made for European and North American voltages or low voltage supplies suitable for aircraft or ambulance requirements. For portable applications there may be an internal sealed rechargeable battery and a state-of-charge indicator.

12.10 Defibrillation discharge waveforms

As an alternative to the over-damped capacitor discharge waveform so far described, truncated exponential and trapezoidal waveforms are also available in various models of commercial defibrillators.

12.11 Portable defibrillators

A defibrillator may be required in a hurry anywhere within a large hospital or carried to the scene of an incident by paramedical staff trained in its use. The design must be sufficiently light in weight and smooth in its contours that it can be carried by an attendant while running or mounted on an emergency cardiac resuscitation trolley. A typical unit might weigh about 13 kg and contain a bank of 10 rechargeable nickel cadmium cells capable of providing the power for up to 100 shocks each of 320 joules into a 50 ohm load and also of powering the cardioscope for four hours of display. These batteries would take 4 hours to completely recharge and the high voltage capacitor is automatically discharged as a safety precaution after 60 seconds. Charging of the capacitor takes of the order of 7 to 10 seconds to attain an energy of 320 joules, depending on the model.

The weight of another defibrillator fitted with a cardiac pacer, cardio-scope and batteries is 10 kg and the unit has a carrying handle and a smooth plastic case. The batteries will provide power for up to 30 discharges of 360 joules each or 2.5 hours of continuous monitoring or 35 minutes with an illuminated warning to indicate that power remains for either a further 35 minutes of monitoring or six 360 joule discharges. Because a defibrillator may be subjected to relatively rough handling, all the integrated circuits should be soldered in place and the printed circuit boards firmly locked in place and plugs and sockets properly secured.

12.12 Implantable pacer-cardioverter-defibrillator

A new development consists of an implantable device which is able to offer a range of automatically delivered therapies aimed at controlling life-threatening occurrences of ventricular arrhythmias such as ventricular tachycardia or ventricular fibrillation. When the device's sensing electrodes detect the presence of ventricular tachycardia, the system delivers a series of nearly imperceptible 'pacing' electrical pulses designed to restore normal sinus rhythm. Only if this approach is ineffective does the device proceed to deliver a defibrillation pulse. It is suggested by the manufacturer that in approximately 90% of ventricular tachycardia episodes the pacing sequence terminated the arrhythmias. It was found that after one year, users of the device experienced a nearly 99% survival from a sudden cardiac death. The defibrillation energy used is of the order of 20 joules. The system uses an epicardial lead system and represented a very sophisticated version of a fully implantable electronic device.

12.13 External pacemaker

When a defibrillator fitted with cardiac-pacing circuitry is switched to the pacer mode, a series of current pulses is available to pace the heart via connection to an anterior-posterior pair of self-adhesive disposable pacing electrodes. Both the pacing rate and stimulus intensity can be set using manual front-panel controls. A typical pacing-rate range might be 30 to 180 beats per minute with a stimulating current range of 0 to 140 mA. The use of external cardiac pacemakers is also covered in Chapter 6.

12.14 Cardiac balloon pumps

When a patient is suffering from an inadequate cardiac output on a temporary basis, perhaps while drug therapy is used to restore myocardial contractility, the pumping action of the left ventricle can be augmented by means of a cardiac balloon pump. A source of gas such as helium or carbon dioxide under pressure is used to inflate a balloon placed in the aorta below the aortic arch. For an adult, the closed volume of the balloon would typically be 40 cc. The balloon is situated at the distal end of a cardiac catheter which is introduced via a femoral artery with a percutaneous or cut-down approach.

The inflation of the balloon is synchronized to the patient's ECG and the initiation of inflation can be adjusted in the cardiac cycle. A safety-bleed valve opens if an inflation pressure of 200 mmHg is exceeded. An alarm is also given if there is a gas loss of more than 5 cc per inflation.

Pumping can continue from one day to a week with an infusion of heparin as an anti-coagulant. If pumping is stopped for a period, the balloon should be inflated manually by means of a syringe about once every 30 minutes to prevent the clotting of blood in the folds of the deflated balloon. In addition to operating from the mains power supply, balloon pumps can operate from the 24 volt supply of an aircraft and have their own battery supply for use during a power failure or when a patient is being moved. Nurses familiar with the technique of balloon pumping will be in a position to reassure patients on whom the device is being used.

Endoscopic equipment

13

13.1 Introduction

The use of both rigid and flexible endoscopes has made possible the viewing of a wide range of body cavities and passages. This has opened up new vistas in terms of the confirmation of a diagnosis and allowed the use of non-invasive or minimally invasive therapeutic procedures. In turn this has expedited the role of day surgery and investigations, with the consequent saving of the cost of an overnight stay in an acute hospital bed and the minimizing of the resulting inconvenience caused to the patient and relatives. Thus, modern endoscopes have done much to aid medicine and surgery and represent a cost-effective use of advances made in optics, light sources and miniature colour television technology.

Endoscopes are used by a variety of clinicians including gastroenterologists, chest physicians, and general, urological, thoracic and orthopaedic surgeons. The instruments are sophisticated and relatively expensive. Nurses are often involved in their disinfection and storage. Handling an electronic or video-endoscopy system requires care and consideration or irreparable damage may be done. An understanding of the technology involved, the advantages it brings to both the patient and clinician and the need to handle delicate components with care should enable nursing staff to work comfortably as part of a multi-disciplinary team using the various forms of endoscopes.

13.2 Direct viewing fibrescopes

Fibrescopes are usually direct viewing, flexible endoscopes which by means of a steerable distal tip can be inserted via the nose, mouth, rectum or urethra. The appropriate designs serve as gastroscopes, duodenoscopes, colonoscopes or bronchoscopes. White light from a source such as a 300 watt xenon semi-flash lamp located outside the patient is transmitted down one bundle of 'incoherent' fibres and via a diverging lens mounted at the distal tip of the fibrescope illuminates the selected site within the patient's body. Light reflected back is collected by a second 'coherent' bundle of fibres and returns to the viewing eyepiece at the proximal end of the fibrescope adjacent to the operator's controls which allow the moveable section at the distal end of the fibrescope to be bent up or down, and left or right, by means of an arrangement of wire cables, Figure 13.1. The fibrescope may have a total length of up to 1.6 metres depending on the clinical application and also contains an instrument channel down which can be passed a biopsy forceps or therapeutic devices plus, in gastroenterological instruments, channels for an irrigating flush of sterile water and an air flow for organ distortion, Figure 13.2.

The operator observes the image directly by means of an eyepiece containing the necessary lenses which are colour corrected and anti-reflection coated. It is possible to clip on a small television camera in order that the image can be displayed on a colour television monitor, for example, for teaching purposes or for showing to a patient. The xenon lamp source of illumination can also be operated under microprocessor control in flash mode for use with endo-photography to enable the image viewed to be captured using a 35 mm reflex camera or a polaroid camera. A typical maximum flash cycling time of one second is possible.

13.2.1 Coherent and non-coherent fibre optic bundles and plates

A fibre optic or 'light pipe' uses the principle of total internal reflection. A fibre optic bundle is constructed from a number of identical flexible glass fibres, each consisting of a central core of one glass surrounded by an outer cladding made from another glass which has a lower value of refractive index than of the glass used for the core.

When a ray of light passes across the interface from one transparent medium to another which is optically more dense, the path of the ray is deflected. Consider a block of glass which has a refractive index n.

Figure 13.1 Fibre Optic Gastroscope. (Courtesy Keymed Ltd.)

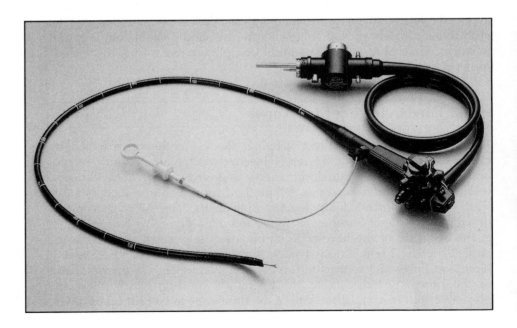

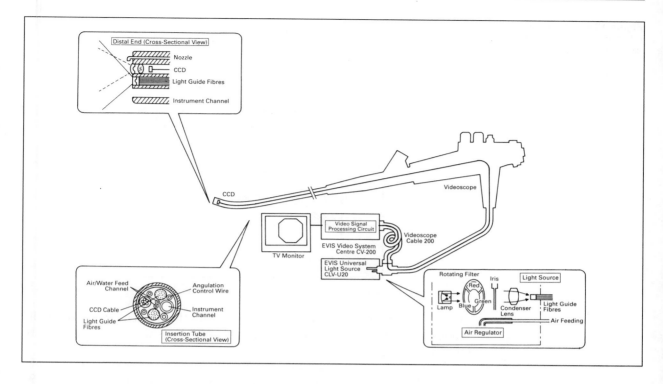

Figure 13.2 Cross-section of a
fibre optic gastroscope.
(Courtesy Keymed Ltd.)

Suppose that a ray of light strikes the front surface of the block making an angle of incidence i between the incident ray and the normal (a line perpendicular to the interface at the point of incidence). Some of the incident light is reflected back into the first block and some is refracted on into the second block at an angle of refraction r to the normal, Figure 13.3. Snell's Law of Refraction is expressed by the relationship $\sin i / \sin r = n$.

Figure 13.3 Reflection and refraction of a ray of light incident on an air-glass interface.

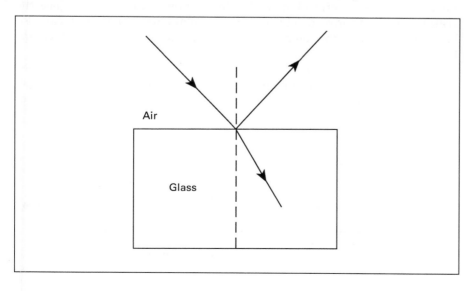

Figure 13.4 Total internal
reflection occurring at an
air/glass interface.

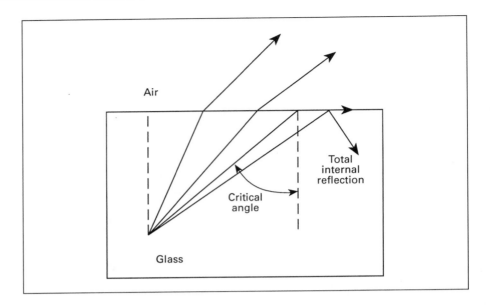

Figure 13.4 Total internal reflection occurring at an air/glass interface.

The constant n has a value which depends on the particular pair of media concerned (in this case air and glass). It is known as the refractive index of that glass with respect to air.

As the angle of incidence is increased there is a corresponding increase, linked by Snell's Law, of the angle of refraction r until when r = 90 degrees all of the incident light is reflected along the interface. At greater angles of incidence, the interface acts as a perfect mirror and all of the light is reflected, Figure 13.4.

For simplicity, the principle of total internal reflection has been described in terms of the interface between air and glass. The angle of incidence at which total internal reflection occurs and there is no refracted ray is known as the critical angle. For the combination of air and glass the critical angle is approximately 40 degrees. Total internal reflection can also be made to occur at the interface between two different types of glass, one having a higher value of refractive index than the other.

In the case of the optical fibre, one end is polished flat and light directed on to it via a suitable lens. By means of a series of multiple internal reflections light is efficiently transmitted down the fibre, Figure 13.5. A number

Figure 13.5 A ray of light undergoing multiple internal reflection while transversing an optical fibre.

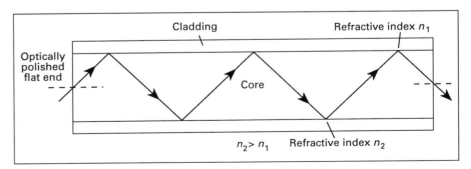

of such fibres can be held within an outer plastic sheath and used to transmit light as in the case of a fibre optic oximeter used *in vivo* to monitor arterial blood-oxygen saturation. This type of bundle is non-coherent and is not used for the viewing of images. The position of the end of any particular fibre need not be precisely the same at both the distal and proximal ends of the bundle.

To conduct images via a coherent fibre bundle each fibre should appear in exactly the same spatial position at both the proximal and distal ends. Consequently, great care must be taken during manufacture to align precisely the position of each individual fibre at the two ends of the bundle. A coherent fibre-optic bundle can be used for viewing images as part of a fibrescope with light from the light source being transmitted to the distal end of the fibrescope via one or two non-coherent bundles.

Over their working life, both inside a patient and during cleaning and disinfection, fibrescopes are subjected to considerable flexing which may eventually cause fibres to fracture. This will gradually degrade the quality of the observed images from a coherent bundle as individual fibres cease to transmit light back from the distal end. Thus, while adequate cleaning of the fibrescope and its channels from debris such as tissue, mucus and faecal material together with appropriate disinfection is essential, fibrescopes should be handled as gently and considerately as possible and not dropped from wet hands! Storage cabinets are available to hold a number of flexible endoscopes vertically in a secure fashion.

13.2.2 Video endoscopes

Fibrescopes have the smallest possible external diameter allowing for the fact that instrument and irrigation channels must also be built into the insertion tube. This is important where the smallest possible diameters are required for paediatric studies. However, there is the problem of image degradation owing to broken fibres and the fibrescope is basically intended for direct viewing by the operator.

These considerations have led to the development of a range of so-called videoscopes in which a miniature television camera 'chip' is mounted at the distal end of the endoscope. Because of the need to make the camera as small as possible a black-and-white sensor may be used, the signal from which is transmitted by a cable back down the endoscope to a video processor control unit and light source. In this, a rotating disk carries three optical filters, one for each primary colour red, green and blue. These are placed in the path of the illumination generated by a xenon lamp. The rotating filters generate three sequential images, red, green and blue, which are fed to the three guns of a colour television tube to display a full colour version of the image as seen by the videoscope. Provision is also available to freeze a particular image free from colour distortion, i.e. there is no separation of the three original primary colour images. An automatically controlled iris is arranged to monitor the peak brightness of the image and by means of the diaphragm to adjust this to prevent overloading of the video system and the resulting 'white-out' of the image.

Electronic magnification, typically times two, is available when a detailed examination of microscopic structures is necessary.

A typical video gastroscope would provide a forward-looking (120 degree) field of view with a depth of field from 3 to 100 mm. The working length is 1.03 metres and the total length 1.33 metres so that it is convenient to have a storage cupboard which will hold a number of flexible endoscopes vertically in a secure fashion. The outer diameter would typically be 10.5 mm and there is a 2.8 mm diameter instrument channel. Biopsy forceps can be used down this channel and are visible at a minimum distance of 4 mm from the distal end of the endoscope. The permissable ambient temperature range is 10–40 degrees Celsius at a relative humidity of 30% to 85% and an ambient pressure range of 525 to 795 mmHg. Typical outside diameters for a videoduodenoscope and a videocolonoscope/sigmoidoscope are respectively 13 mm and 15.4 mm. Circular plates of fibre optic fibres are used as an efficient method of coupling together electro-optical devices, e.g. an X-ray image intensifier to its associated television camera, as in a mobile X-ray image intensifier used during hip-pinning procedures in orthopaedic surgery.

13.2.3 Complete television endoscopy systems

For use in endoscopy and day-surgery units, a complete television endoscopy system usually comprises two trolleys connected by a multi-way cable. The first carries the light source, television-control unit and a keyboard with which to enter patient and image-identification data. All the controls are touch sensitive and can easily be wiped over for cleaning and disinfection. The second trolley carries the image monitor mounted at a convenient viewing height, a video recorder for storing the television-format images and a hard-copy device. This could be a high quality colour television monitor whose image can be photographed by an attached 35 mm camera fitted with a remote release switch. Alternatively, it could be a video printer using the principle of thermotransfer and utilizing the three primary colours red, green and blue each in 256 shades. The time required to print a full three-colour image is 80 seconds.

A built-in mains-isolation transformer for use with all the components of the system, except the xenon light source, limits the magnitude of the leakage currents to conform to international standards. The trolleys are fitted with large diameter casters and brakes for ease of movement, Figure 13.6.

13.2.4 Endo-therapy accessories

Once a visual examination of the chosen site within the body has been completed it is often possible to insert into the instrument channel of the endoscope a suitable accessory to enable therapy to be performed. A wide range of accessories is available including: biopsy forceps, grasping forceps, cautery electrodes, cutting loops for the treatment of tumours and wire-basket devices for the extraction of calculi, surgical scissors, cytology brush and a biliary drainage tube.

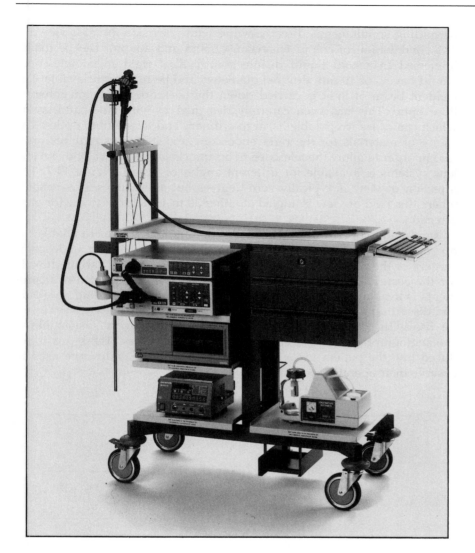

Figure 13.6 Trolley-mounted video endoscopy system. (Courtesy Keymed Ltd.)

13.3 Rigid endoscopes

Laparoscopes are extensively employed in minimally invasive diagnostic and therapeutic procedures within the body. The rigid metal telescope is passed into the body cavity concerned via a metal or plastic cannula which has been passed through the skin and underlying tissue via an opening made with a metal trocar having a pyramidal tip.

The same xenon light source from a particular manufacturer can be used with his range of fibrescopes, video endoscopes and rigid endoscopes. A high resolution 'chip' type of miniature colour television camera can be either directly coupled to a rigid endoscope or via an optical beam splitter permitting simultaneous direct viewing with television-monitor viewing. The combination of colour television camera and adaptor can be totally immersed in a cold liquid disinfectant. Typical rigid metal telescopes would have 5 or 10 mm external diameters and be fully autoclavable. The incident beam of light is carried down the telescope via a non-coherent fibre optic. This has been carefully designed to withstand autoclaving which can cause irreparable harm to ordinary endoscope fibre optics. The choice of materials for the rigid endoscope and its lenses requires great care in order to allow the telescope to be autoclaved. A choice of distal end lens systems is available for different angles of vision, Figure 13.7. The direction of view is typically zero degrees but alternatives are available where this field of view is angled at either 30 to 45 degrees to the forward direction.

Rigid endoscopes are used with insufflators and pumps to enable the operator to control the use of suction or irrigation during endoscopic surgery or the use of a 9-litres-per-minute high gas flow of carbon dioxide for the accurate control of pneumoperitoneum. A wide range of instruments is available for use down the rigid endoscope including: grasping and dissecting forceps, hook and straight scissors, electrodes, a laser insert for use with 600 micrometre surgical laser light delivery system fibres, cholangiography clamp, needle holders and retractors. These are introduced into the patient via a second aperture and the endoscope used to observe their operation.

Figure 13.7 Light transmission in a rigid endoscope and lens system. (Courtesy Keymed Ltd.)

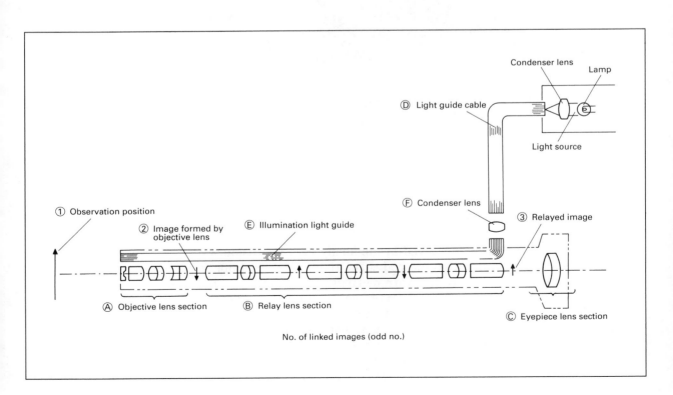

13.3.1 Rigid endoscopes for thoracoscopy

Diagnostic thoracoscopy allows direct observation of the interior of the thorax and for intra-thoracic tissue biopsy. Therapeutic thoracoscopy has application in areas such as the removal of haematoma and ablation of pleural empyema. Muscle tissue is first severed using surgical diathermy, a blunt trocar used to make a suitable opening into the pleural cavity followed by a rigid trocar tube through which is passed a rigid metal telescope which can be autoclaved at 134 degrees Celsius. A heater unit is available for the pre-heating of telescopes to body temperature in order to minimize the tendency for a telescope to fog when it is introduced into the thoracic cavity. A range of accessories such as forceps, scissors and diathermy electrodes is available for use during thoracoscopy.

13.4 Surgical lasers for use during endoscopy

Laser laparoscopy makes use of a flexible fibre, often of quartz, to guide a powerful beam of single wavelength (monochromatic) light, from a surgical laser, down a suitable laparoscope to remove tissue or to seal bleeding points. Laser light is also coherent, unlike light emitted from an ordinary lamp. That is to say, all the constituent light-energy particles or 'photons' travel in time and in space in phase with each other. They form a wavefront. The laser-generated beam of light is well-collimated, i.e. it exhibits very little divergence or spreading out. The combination of monochromaticity, coherence and collimation enables a beam of laser light to be focused very precisely to a sharp spot of energy to interact with tissue.

Lasers used include neodymium-YAG and holmium-YAG which emit in the near infra-red (Nd-YAG at 1.06 micrometres, holmium-YAG at 2.1 micrometres) and carbon dioxide which emits at 10.6 micrometres. These wavelengths are too long to be visible and so an auxiliary helium-neon laser is provided to generate a visible aiming beam of red light. A solid-state Nd-YAG surgical laser, Figure 13.8, would typically generate a maximum output power at tissue of 60 watts and the helium-neon laser would have a 5 milli-watt output.

It is possible to adjust the length of the exposure time and the length of the interval before the next exposure over the range from 0.5 seconds exposure followed by an interval of 0.3 seconds to 0.1 seconds exposure followed by an interval of 0.4 seconds. The light output of the laser is transmitted down the instrument channel of the endoscope via a Teflon-coated quartz glass fibre which has a diameter of 0.2 mm, 0.4 mm or 0.6 mm. Fibres can be supplied with special tips which make possible direct contact with tissue and precisely defined incisions. Lammer, J., Pilger, E., Decrinis, M., Quehenberger, F., Klein, G. and Stark, G. (1992) 'Pulsed excimer laser versus continuous Nd:YAG laser versus conventional angio-plasty of peripheral arterial occlusions: prospective, controlled, randomised trial', *The Lancet*, **340**, 1183–8 used a Neodymium-Yag laser

Figure 13.8 Neodymium-YAG
surgical laser.
(Courtesy Keymed Ltd.)

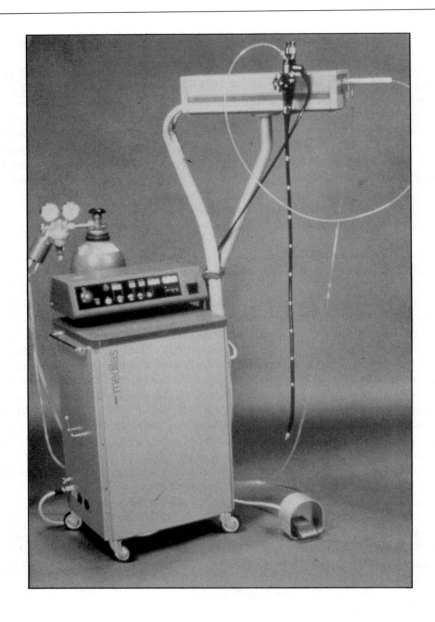

with a single 2.2 mm single (600 micrometre) fibre fitted with a 'sapphire'
contact probe having a spherical configuration.

Quartz glass fibres cannot be used with the longer wavelength output of
a continuous wave carbon dioxide laser. Here, a hollow, straight 'air' fibre
is used which has a typical inner opening diameter of 1.2 mm and an
external diameter of 3.05 mm with a length of either 30 or 45 cm. The fibre
is continuously purged with carbon dioxide gas at a flow rate in the range
0.5 to 1 litre per minute in order to protect the delivery system from

possible contamination from vaporized tissue. Flexible fibres for use with carbon dioxide lasers are not yet available.

13.4.1 Safety precautions with surgical lasers

Lasers generate intense beams of well-collimated monochromatic light which can travel for long distances. It is clearly important not to look directly into a beam of laser light because of the damage which is highly likely to result to the eye. Laser light is easily reflected and scattered and it is this source of laser light which is likely to catch staff, such as nurses, unawares. Laser light, in a well-designed laser system, should be confined within the boundary enclosure of the laser and its delivery system. Light emerging from the delivery system can pose a risk to the laser operator and to associated staff in the room if commonsense precautions have not been taken.

With lasers which generate an output in the visible region of the spectrum, such as helium-neon or argon lasers, it is vital to have a safety mechanism automatically in place to reduce the beam power to a safe level in order that any back-scattered radiation which returns to the observing operator's eye cannot cause damage. Lasers such as Nd-YAG, holmium-YAG and carbon dioxide generate invisible infra-red radiation, and care must be taken to check that no leaks can arise in the delivery system as stray radiation can burn clothing on a person standing back several feet from the laser. All medical laser systems should be checked on a regular basis by a laser safety adviser and used by a trained and competent operator.

The January 1992 issue of *Health Devices* indicates that like surgical diathermy, a surgical laser can set surgical drapes on fire. Immediately after each use, the laser should be put into the stand-by mode in order to prevent accidental operation. The laser can burn through the endotracheal tube which is usually full of an anaesthetic gas mixture containing oxygen – with disastrous results for the patient. Laser-resistant endotracheal tubes are obtainable which are more or less effective according to the January 1992 issue of *Health Devices*. The manufacturers recommend that the tube's cuff should be filled with saline rather than air. Cotton gauze sponges (pledgets) soaked in saline can be packed round the endotracheal tube to protect it from the laser beam.

13.5 Angiofibrescopes

Fibre optic angioscopes are a development of fibreoptic endoscopes. They are inserted into the patient's vasculature by one of two methods. In the first, the angioscope is inserted percutaneously as with a conventional catheter. In the second, the angioscope is inserted directly into the vessel through an incision made into the exposed vessel. The angiologist may choose to make use of a sheath introducer or a guide catheter may be inserted into the sheath introducer and the angioscope then inserted into the catheter. To ensure a clear field of view it is necessary to keep blood from the site. This can be accomplished by flushing sterile saline solution through the space existing between the angioscope and the sheath introducer or guide catheter.

In one form of angiofibrescope the outer diameter is 2.2 mm and the distal tip can be angulated by plus or minus 120 degrees. The field of view is 75 degrees in the forward direction (0 degrees) with a depth of field from 2 to 50 mm. The working length of the Teflon-covered insertion section is 1 metre and the total length is 3.33 metres. There is a 1 mm channel for irrigation purposes. The fibre optic light guide is ring-shaped in section to provide an even illumination across the full viewing field. The angiofibrescope can be sterilized in ethylene oxide gas or cold fluid.

Versions of angiofibrescope are available with an outside diameter as small as 0.8 mm giving a 55 degree field of view and a depth of field of 1 to 50 mm. The working length is 1.3 metres and the total length is 3.5 metres. Angiofibrescopes are used for the confirmation and analysis of atheroma, thrombus and calcification. Endo-therapy devices available for use in conjunction with angiofibrescopes include valvulotomes for the disruption of the venous valves in the lower limbs and grasping forceps for the retrieval of thrombi, residual venous valves or flaps. A thumb ring allows single-handed operation of the device even when the associated insertion tube is significantly curved.

13.6 Sterilization and disinfection of endoscopes and accessories

Sterilizing an instrument will render it germ free in contrast to disinfection which will kill off any pathogenic micro-organisms which are present. Sterilization is effected by means of autoclaving or the use of ethylene oxide gas or formalin vapour in suitable protective cabinets. Sterilization can also be obtained by the use of glutaraldehyde which is normally used to disinfect endoscopes. For sterilization of resistant pathogenic spores, including *Clostridium tetani*, complete immersion in gluteraldehyde solution is required. In contrast for disinfection and terminal decontamination, immersion for a minimum of 10 minutes will destroy vegetative pathogens such as *Pseudomonas aeruginosa* and viruses such as hepatitis B and HIV on inanimate surfaces, while immersion for 1 hour is required for the destruction of *Mycobacterium tuberculosis*.

Although rigid metal endoscopes are available which can be sterilized without harm by autoclaving, this procedure would damage flexible endoscopes based on the use of conventional fibre optics. Flexible endoscopes are designed, with the exception of their channels, to be impervious to water and thus a video endoscope or fibrescope can be totally immersed in a liquid disinfectant solution such as glutaraldehyde. Air pressure leakage detectors are available to check for the presence of pinhole-size leaks in a flexible endoscope in order to minimize the incidence of damage to the interior of an endoscope due to the ingress of water. Ethylene oxide gas in an enclosed chamber is also suitable but glutaraldehyde disinfection is convenient in that it can be accomplished relatively close to the endoscopy room and in times sufficiently short as to be compatible with a busy list in conjunction with the alternation of endoscopes. Cleaning/disinfection times of 10–15 minutes are feasible.

Prior to disinfection, pre-cleaning is accomplished by wiping the distal insertion tube with gauze. After checking for leaks, cleaning is performed by immersing and washing an immersible endoscope in cleaning solution. Any debris which has accumulated in the endoscope or its accessories needs to be removed by using suitable cleaning brushes to brush out the entire suction line of the endoscope. The suction and biopsy valves are washed and any debris removed with a toothbrush. Finally, water and air are alternately aspirated through the channel several times. Gross deposits of debris can be removed by conventional washing, but ultrasonic cleaning is required to clean endoscopic accessories such as biopsy forceps. A built-in heater for the waterbath of the ultrasonic cleaner softens debris which has become hardened and assists in cleaning entrapped debris from between the coils of sheathed accessories. The metal baskets into which the accessories are placed for cleaning are designed to properly coil the biopsy forceps in order to avoid damaging the sheath. The vibration and fluid cavitation generated by the ultrasonic transducer dislodge the debris. Without proper cleaning endoscopes may not be properly disinfected. Proteinaceous material becomes fixed to endoscope surfaces by the aldehyde of the gluteraldehyde, which is why a preliminary cleaning is essential.

Both manual, semi-automatic and fully automatic systems for disinfecting endoscopes with glutaraldehyde are available. Three fluids are involved: water rinse, detergent and glutaraldehyde. Recommendations for suitable procedures are contained in the paper 'Cleaning and disinfection of equipment for gastrointestinal flexible endoscopy: interim recommendations of a Working Party of the British Society of Gastroenterology', *Gut*, August 1988, **29**, 1134–51. The minimum cycle time is normally taken to be 15 minutes which includes a 4-minute exposure to the glutaraldehyde. Automatic and semi-automatic systems include electric pumps to change the various fluids. Care is required when irrigating the endoscope channels to provide a high fluid flow rate without the development of high pressures which could damage the endoscope.

The fully automatic system is plumbed-in like a washing machine and the glutaraldehyde is discharged directly into a drain. Manual and semi-automatic systems are trolley mounted, Figure 13.9, and care must be taken to minimize the inhalation of glutaraldehyde vapour in filling and emptying the lidded chamber which holds the endoscope.

In the UK the Health and Safety Commission has adopted a ten-minute time-weighted average occupational exposure limit of 0.2 parts per million for glutaraldehyde which requires that disinfection of endoscopes should not be performed in 'open' systems (Department of Health, *Safety Action Bulletin No. 81*, March 1992 'Glutaraldehyde disinfectants – use and

Figure 13.9 Semi-automatic glutaraldehyde sterilization system for use with flexible endoscopes and their accessories. (Courtesy Safelab Systems Ltd.)

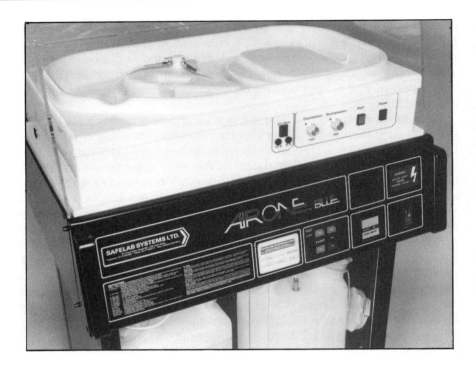

Figure 13.10 Active carbon filter for use with a semi-automatic endoscope disin-fector. (Courtesy Keymed Ltd.)

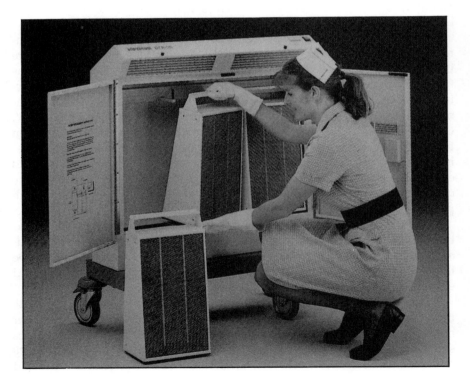

management'). The vapour can be irritating. Skin contact should be avoided by the use of protective clothing, such as rubber gloves, boots, over-apron and eye goggles.

An add-on disinfectant fume extractor based on the use of active carbon filters is available to absorb glutaraldehyde vapour emission from manual and semi-automatic systems, but other types of system have a built-in carbon filter, Figure 13.10. Room air is drawn in through the front opening of the plastic cabinet and sweeps issuing vapour through the filter. After absorption of vapour the cleaned air is vented to the room away from the operator via the back of the cabinet.

In order to minimize corrosion to objects immersed in glutaraldehyde solution the pH of the solution should be pH 7 or above and corrosion inhibitors are added. Rubber, plastic, nickel, chromium plate, stainless steel, carbon steel, copper, brass and aluminium should not be harmed (Miner, N. A., McDowell, J. W., Willcockson, G. W., Bruckner, N. I., Stark, R. L. and Whitmore, J. (1977) 'Antimicrobial and other properties of a new stabilised alkaline glutaraldehyde disinfectant/steriliser', *American Journal of Hospital Pharmacy*, **34**, 376–82).

Safety Action Bulletin SAB(92)1, January 1992 from the Medical Devices Directorate of the UK's Department of Health draws attention to the fact that in addition to routine preventative maintenance, all tanks and fluid pathways forming part of endoscope washer/disinfectors must be regularly drained, cleaned and disinfected to minimize the possibility of re-contamination of the endoscope.

14 Surgical Diathermy Units

14.1 Introduction

Surgical diathermy units of various types are widely encountered in operating rooms. In North America they are known as electrosurgery units. They are essentially powerful radio transmitters and usually cause significant interference to the tracings on patient monitors and recorders. In some cases it may be possible to limit the bandwidth of the patient-monitor channels to allow, for example, the viewing of a basic ECG and foregoing the quality of a full diagnostic ECG during the operation of the diathermy. The interference can damage mechanical devices such as pen recorders owing to the mains-frequency modulation of the radiofrequency causing large excursions of the pen arm. It may be necessary to switch off devices of this nature when the diathermy is to be operated. There is also the possibility of diathermy units causing burns to the patient and setting the drapes alight. Hence vigilance is important when diathermy is used.

A monopolar surgical diathermy unit basically consists of a radiofrequency transmitter whose active output terminal is connected to a cutting needle electrode mounted in an insulating handpiece. The other, indifferent, terminal is connected to a large area of flexible neutral metal plate electrode (typically 150 sq cm) placed under the patient or wrapped around a thigh. This is also known as the dispersive electrode since it disperses the diathermy current over a large area of skin.

In a radiofrequency earthed type of monopolar diathermy the neutral plate electrode is connected to earth, *not* directly but via a capacitor of such a value of capacitance that it presents a low impedance to earth for the passage of radiofrequency diathermy current and a high impedance to mains-frequency currents. In an isolated monopolar diathermy, both the cutting and plate electrodes are fed from the secondary winding of a well-insulated radiofrequency transformer so that both electrodes are isolated from earth.

In a bipolar type of isolated diathermy unit (bipolar diathermy) neither the active nor the indifferent output terminals are referred to earth, so that there is no connection or components present between the diathermy output and earth. As before, both output terminals are fed from the secondary winding of an output transformer.

For delicate work, for example in neurosurgery, ophthalmology and laparoscopy, bipolar diathermy is often employed. There is now no neutral plate electrode to complete the circuit to the isolated output generator. Specially designed forceps are used with each blade insulated from the other. The radiofrequency current passes down one blade, through the small volume of tissue between the blades and back via the second blade. The close proximity of the tips of the blades minimizes the spread of diathermy current to adjacent patient-monitoring electrodes and hence the risk of burns to the patient. The current density of the radiofrequency current, which is normally activated by operating a footswitch, is sufficiently high that an arc is struck between the tip of the cutting needle and the patient. If the output power chosen is sufficient, the arc can be used for cutting through tissue such as the abdominal wall or dividing internal tissues. In addition to the main output, which is usually a pure sinewave, for cutting tissue alternative power settings and often different waveforms enable the diathermy to be employed for coagulating bleeding points and providing haemostasis. In practice, the sinewave output is arranged to be formed into a series of bursts of sinewaves in order to provide sufficient time to allow for coagulation to occur as the blood cools in the intervals between successive bursts of tissue heating. The diathermy unit is also normally provided with a heavy current low-voltage output at mains frequency which can be used to heat a wire loop for cautery purposes.

14.2 Types of diathermy generator

Surgical diathermy units have to be rugged in construction and reliable in use. They should be sealed against the ingress of blood and irrigation fluids and easily cleaned. The original versions were based on the use of a spark-gap in which the negative resistance associated with the high voltage discharge across a spark-gap was used to set a radiofrequency tuned circuit into oscillation.

Although rugged, the action of the spark discharge superimposes upon the nominal frequency of the tuned circuit a large number of harmonics and noise spikes. This 'dirty' waveform is impossible to filter out from patient monitors and plays havoc with the display of electrophysiological signals. Spark-gap diathermies have very few components to wear out and may still be found in hospitals.

The advent of thermionic valves led to the appearance of simple valve oscillator diathermies in which the valve functions as both a rectifier for the high-voltage a.c. supply and as part of the oscillator circuit. The radio-frequency output is 100% modulated at the mains frequency and the presence of this substantial 50 Hz component (60 Hz in North America) plays havoc with patient-monitor displays and can easily damage pen recorders.

A better arrangement employs full-wave rectification for the high-voltage supply to the valve oscillator circuit and uses filters to ensure that the diathermy output is a clean sinewave at about 1.75 MHz which is much more easily filtered out in patient monitors. Assuming a patient load of 150 ohms, a typical valve diathermy set would have a maximum output power of 400 watts available for cutting tissue. For cutting with coagulation, the output waveform can be changed to be bursts of 1.75 MHz at selectable repetition rates of 50 Hz, 20 kHz or 60 kHz.

The current versions of surgical diathermy units are all solid-state systems based on the use of transistors rather than spark-gaps or valves and operate at a frequency of no higher than 500 kHz. A typical unit would provide a maximum output of 350 to 400 watts pure radiofrequency into a 200 ohm load for cutting with the output isolated from earth and a reduced power output of 80 to 150 watts for coagulation, a 300 watt pulsed monopolar (neutral plate connected to earth via a capacitor) output for cutting with coagulation, and a bipolar output of 15 to 50 watts for delicate work, Figure 14.1.

Figure 14.1 Eschmann Model TD 411RS Electrosurgical equipment. The maximum power output is 400 watts into a 200 ohm load at a frequency of 475 kHz. (Courtesy Eschmann Brothers & Walsh Ltd.)

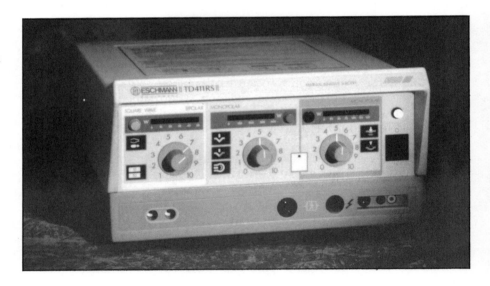

14.3 Contact/continuity plate electrode monitoring circuits

British Standard 5724 Part Two 'Medical electrical equipment: specification for high frequency surgical equipment (1983)' requires that radiofrequency earthed (monopolar) diathermy sets, providing in excess of 50 watts rated output power, must have a circuit to monitor the continuity of the neutral plate electrode and its connecting cable which will produce an audible alarm and switch off the diathermy power if a break occurs in the cable. A twin-core cable is used in order to provide a continuous electrical circuit to and from the plate.

It must be remembered that this alarm circuit will not monitor the effectiveness of the contact between the plate and the patient or that the plate is in position on the patient. Monopolar-type diathermies having an isolated output do not need to have a neutral plate electrode alarm fitted. However, it is important that the neutral plate electrode of an isolated output diathermy cannot attain a high radiofrequency voltage. This situation could arise if contact between the plate and the patient was poor or if the active electrode came into contact with an earthed metal object while the diathermy was in use.

Some isolated output diathermies are provided with a neutral plate electrode monitoring circuit which will detect a rise in the voltage of the plate and terminate the diathermy output if the plate voltage exceeds a preset limit, typically about 100 volts. An alternative approach is to monitor the radiofrequency current leaving the diathermy unit and also that returning to it via the neutral plate lead. The main component of any difference in the currents arises from currents flowing from the patient and the diathermy wiring to earth. When this difference current exceeds a preset value it is arranged that the diathermy output is automatically terminated.

14.4 Hazards from surgical diathermy units

14.4.1 Hazards to patient monitoring equipment

If there is mains-frequency modulation present on the radiofrequency output of the diathermy, the modulation will affect patient monitors and can block out the electrophysiological signals and can damage mechanical components such as pen recorders. Patient monitors designed for use in operating rooms are fitted with a filter which can be switched in to limit the frequency response of the monitor, typically to 40 Hz, in order to minimize upset to the tracings.

14.4.2 Burns to the patient

Burns due to overheating of the electrode can occur when the plate electrode makes poor contact with the patient. Radiofrequency power causes heating in the relatively high contact resistance.

A more subtle problem occurs with the production of radiofrequency burns (which are slow to heal) under electrodes connected to the patient, typically ECG electrodes. Such burns arise when there is a fault with the plate electrode (electrode not in place or the connecting cable broken). Radiofrequency current then finds its way back to earth via the input impedance of the signal (ECG) amplifier and the resulting current density under the small area ECG electrode is sufficient to cause the formation of a burn. Similarly, a faulty plate electrode can allow diathermy current to flow to earth via a part of the patient, perhaps a finger, which either touches an earthed trolley or is close to it when the diathermy unit is activated. The diathermy current can pass through the capacitance formed by the finger, airgap and trolley. Burns have been reported at the site of oesophageal and rectal temperature probes due to localized points of contact with surrounding tissue.

Similar considerations apply to the use of monopolar diathermy with a metallic orthopaedic implant situated in tissue between the active and indifferent electrodes of the diathermy. There are not many reports of internal damage to tissue in the vicinity of orthopaedic implants because the damage caused is not readily visible.

Thermal injury to tissue can result when the temperature of the tissue is caused to exceed for a sufficient time the threshold of 45 degrees Celsius for protein denaturation. During electrosurgery, such injuries occur when the diathermy current is confined to a small surface area during activation of the diathermy. Current densities of approximately 100 mA r.m.s. per square centimetre or more will damage tissue. It is possible that current densities of about 50 mA r.m.s. per square centimetre may not damage well-perfused tissue but bone and poorly perfused tissue are at risk.

Monopolar diathermy current can be confined to a small cross-sectional area deep within tissue where metallic prosthetic devices are located between the active and plate electrodes. This can occur particularly with plate implants and intra-medullary locking nails where screws may protrude beyond the main portion of the prosthesis and high current densities arise at the tips of the screws. Wherever possible, bipolar diathermy should be used in the presence of metallic implants to localize current spread. If this is not feasible then the monopolar active and plate electrodes should be sited so that the implant does not lie between them.

14.4.3 Fires and explosions

Great care must be exercised to ensure that sparks from a diathermy cannot ignite methane in bowel gases or an oxygen/cyclopropane/ether anaesthetic mixture, as the resulting explosion may well have fatal consequences. Inadvertent operation of a diathermy unit can cause a fire by igniting spirit-soaked surgical drapes.

14.4.4 Diathermy hazards to patients fitted with a cardiac pacemaker

When monopolar surgical diathermy is employed, and the tissue between the cutting needle electrode and the plate electrode contains an implanted cardiac pacemaker and its connecting leads, there is a risk that the operation of the pacemaker may be affected by the diathermy current or that burns may occur at the implantation site of the pacing lead. The risk to pacing will be much less from a bipolar diathermy because of the highly localized current path between the forceps-type electrodes.

14.4.5 Danger to the diathermy operator

The higher output voltages required from diathermy units to produce 'spray' discharges for sealing an area of tissue can puncture surgical gloves and shock the operator if inadequate insulation exists as part of the electrodes.

Bipolar diathermy units are used in conjunction with an endoscope, the diathermy catheter containing the pair of conductors being passed down a channel of the endoscope. The localized spread of the diathermy current, together with the plastic covering of the endoscope and the eyepiece made of plastic, prevent the operator from being at risk when the diathermy is operated.

14.4.6 Mechanical problems with surgical diathermy sets

The footswitch is particularly vulnerable to the ingress of blood, saline or water from washing the floor. The connecting cables can suffer damage from the impact of trolleys. Pneumatic-type footswitches are sometimes used to overcome the problems associated with electrical versions.

Nearly all operating rooms contain a surgical diathermy unit. A feeling of familiarity should not be allowed to blind operating-room staff to the hazards which may occur when the diathermy or cautery is used. Regular maintenance should be undertaken by the supplier.

14.4.7 The use of square waveforms

Some diathermy unit manufacturers are providing a square wave rather than a sinewave output on the grounds that for the same power a higher voltage sinewave is needed and this increases the amount of thermal necrosis caused to tissue. A blended output based on a modulated square wave is used in minimally invasive procedures to provide effective cutting of tissue with adequate haemostasis. The diathermy set is designed to operate with the blend output into a low tissue resistance of approximately 80 to 100 ohms since the electrical resistance of the tissue changes markedly with cutting and coagulation. For example, in laparoscopic cholecystectomy, maximum haemostasis is needed during excision and dissection but with minimal tissue necrosis and tissue adhesion.

Dessication is needed for coagulation and the diathermy is now required to produce a high flow of current in order to seal both arterial and venous vessels in a variety of types of tissue where the load resistance is varying. Desiccation is achieved by applying localized heating to the end of the blood vessel concerned which causes the vessel to contract and eventually occlude. This takes several seconds depending on the thermal mass involved. The use of a square wave reduces arcing at the start and finish of the wave because of the rapid rise and fall times of the output pulse and thus limits unnecessary tissue damage.

Fulguration (cutting under water) is a mode of diathermy used when excising tissue from within a fluid-filled bladder. A higher voltage square wave is employed to allow a diathermy spark to be initiated even with a conducting medium such as sterile saline used for bladder irrigation. Better tissue penetration of the coagulation is claimed which is required in trans-urethral prostatectomy.

15 | Patient Safety

15.1 Introduction

Underlying the use of medical instrumentation of all sorts must be the principle of ensuring at all times the safety of both the patients concerned and the associated staff. Much equipment is powered from the electrical mains and hence poses the hazards of electric shock and, in extreme cases, of electrocution. Both static and current electricity can initiate fires and explosions in the presence of suitable flammable agents and both direct and alternating current power supplies can give rise to burns.

The hazard of cross-infection between patients can arise when relatively expensive items such as blood-pressure transducers, ventilators, endoscopes and incubators have to be used in succession with a variety of patients. In addition to the risks presented to patients and their closely associated staff, service engineers may be exposed to a risk of infection when they are asked to repair apparatus which has not been properly disinfected or sterilized in accordance with the manufacturer's instructions.

The working environment is important in terms of occupational health, and problems may arise due to excessive discharge of anaesthetic gas and vapour mixtures into an operating room or developer and fixer fumes into X-ray-department dark rooms. Equipment such as compressors may emit oil or vapour fumes to be inhaled by a patient. The mechanical integrity of equipment used with patients must be subject to a regular check. Parts of an equipment may fall off and hit the patient. The headrest of a patient couch may collapse, throwing the patient on to the floor, or a moving part may squash a patient if an end-of-travel microswitch fails to operate.

In the United Kingdom hazards to patients bring an increasing risk of litigation under the requirements of the Health and Safety at Work Act following the removal of Crown Immunity from National Health Service Hospitals. Product-liability legislation can render an individual liable if equipment under his/her control is shown to be in a dangerous condition or is used negligently. The vigilance of the Health and Safety Executive Inspectorate has to be borne in mind. In other countries, particularly those of North America, increasingly severe legal requirements govern the use of equipment with patients.

15.2 Dangers from electric shock

15.2.1 Macroshock at mains frequencies

A macroshock is a gross event which occurs when a patient becomes connected between an electrical conductor at a relatively high voltage such as the 'line' lead of the mains supply and a conductor at a relatively low voltage such as the neutral or earth leads of the mains supply. A classic situation is that of a patient who is touching an earthed water pipe and inadvertently touches the metal case of an electrical appliance which is not earthed due to the occurrence of a fault allowing the case to become 'live'. Depending upon the amount of current flowing, the victim of an electric shock may feel nothing untoward, feel a slight tingling sensation, be unable to let go of the 'live' object, suffer from severe muscular spasm, become apnoeic, go into ventricular fibrillation or suffer serious burns. The threshold value for sensation and the more serious effect increases with increasing frequency.

At values of current smaller than the 'hold-on' value it is possible for the patient to let go of the 'live' object with which contact has been made. At higher values of current the resulting muscular spasm makes this impossible, deterioration of the skin occurs at the site of contact and electrocution may occur from the large current which flows through the body.

An average value for the 'hold-on' current at 60 Hz is 10.5 mA for women and 16 mA for men due to the difference in muscular development. For mains-frequency currents passed through the skin via either the upper or lower limbs, the threshold of sensation occurs at approximately 1 mA r.m.s., muscular spasm and paralysis start between 10 to 16 mA and ventricular fibrillation can occur in the region of 70 to 100 mA.

The current density at the heart is important and this will be influenced by the magnitude of the current passing through the body and the sites of entrance and exit. For example, if current passes from arm to arm, only some 3% will pass through the heart, whereas if the current passes from head to feet some 10% passes through the heart.

Much domestic-type electrical equipment is mounted inside a metal case with the case being connected to the earth lead of the three-core mains cable. A typical example would be an electric fan used by the bedside. If a fault in the insulation occurs inside the fan housing and the line lead of the mains comes into contact with the earthed metal case, a short-circuit occurs and the resulting large short-circuit current blows the fuse in the mains 3-pin plug. In British Standard 5724 this type of good quality domestic equipment with a single layer of insulation is designated Type H. It is not intended to be permanently connected to a patient.

Medical electronic equipment which is designed for direct connection to patients is designated Type B. It uses the principle of double insulation and its stray leakage currents into or out from the patient must lie within specified limits under both normal operating and single-fault conditions. A single-fault condition occurs, for example, when only one layer of insulation fails or the line and neutral connections from the equipment to the mains supply become interchanged.

Type B equipment is intended for direct connection to the skin of a patient as with an ECG or EEG amplifier. It uses double insulation and the maximum permitted leakage current at mains frequencies is 100 microamperes under normal operating conditions and 500 microamperes under single-fault conditions. Type B equipment does not have a protective earth lead since it is double insulated from the mains and the external case is anyway often made from non-metallic material. An isolated signal earth input connection can be provided if a differential input is required to a signal amplifier, such as that for the ECG or EEG. This is purely for electrophysiological reference purposes and does not carry possible short-circuit currents to a fuse.

15.2.2 Microshock at mains frequencies

This is a more subtle form of electric shock hazard and occurs when leakage current can flow directly to or from the heart. The connection to the heart is commonly a cardiac pacing catheter with its tip anchored in the right ventricle. A hazard may also be posed in this respect by a saline-filled cardiac catheter with its tip within a cardiac chamber. However, the electrical connection to the heart will not be so definite as with the pacing catheter. Mains-frequency currents of the order of 100 microamperes or more into the human heart can give rise to irregularities in the pumping action which at higher currents may proceed to ventricular fibrillation.

Type CF equipment as defined in British Standard 5724 is designed for use in patients who may have a cardiac pacing lead in place or a pressure catheter in a cardiac chamber. The maximum permitted leakage current under normal operating conditions is 10 microamperes rising to a maximum of 50 microamperes when a single-fault condition occurs. The 'F' designation means that the electrical input to the equipment is fully floating with respect to earth, i.e. that the input terminals are earth-free. This can be accomplished by using a low-voltage battery-powered pre-amplifier separated from the main circuitry via an optical isolator. The pre-amplifier may modulate the light output from a photodiode. The light falls on to a photocell and the electrical output from the photocell is subsequently demodulated to yield a version of the input signal. Thus the only connection between the pre-amplifier and the main amplifier is a beam of light – there is no direct electrical connection.

15.3 Safety of medical electrical systems

The International Electrotechnical Commission was responsible for the philosophy embodied in British Standard 5724 which essentially focuses on individual medical electrical equipments, such as patient monitors. However, there is now an increasing tendency to make use of systems of equipment which can include non-specific medical equipment such as personal computers and video recorders. It is these items, often good quality domestic items, which will not comply with the detailed requirements of BS 5724. Thus, their influence on the safety of the whole system may be crucial.

There are two possible situations obtaining in respect of the electrical safety of a multiple device system. On the one hand, individual components may be operating simultaneously connected at the same time to a patient, but not connected to each other, e.g. ECG and EEG monitors. On the other hand, the items of equipment may be temporarily connected together by the operator, as in the case of video-endoscopy equipment connected to a personal computer, or the two equipments may have been permanently interconnected by the system's supplier.

A new standard is to be released covering 'Medical electrical equipment. Part 1: General requirements for safety. 1. Collateral standard: safety requirements for medical electrical systems.' Electrical Safety Testers are available which make the routine testing of electrical equipment used in intensive care situations a simple procedure. As an example, the Rigel 255 Safety Tester, Figure 15.1, will measure the continuity of the protective earth connection at currents of 1 or 10 amperes, insulation resistance in the range 1 to 100 megohms measured at 500 volts and various currents, such as the earth-leakage current, enclosure-leakage current and patient-leakage current. The tester can also measure the mains voltage at the supply outlet and the current drawn by the equipment. A digital display of the results and a print-out are provided.

An additional aspect of patient safety at mains frequencies involves the security of the mains supply. The hospital's normal mains supply is usually derived from two or more feeder lines, each able to supply the hospital's load, in order to guard against a local failure of the supply. If this does occur, it should be possible to move items by hand, such as the electrically driven patient couch of a major X-ray unit, in order to permit access to the patient. Intensive care locations such as operating rooms, intensive care units and the renal dialysis unit can receive limited power from the hospital's diesel-engine-driven emergency generator which automatically starts up when the normal power supply fails. Smaller items such as an incubator or ventilator can be powered from a non-interruptible a.c. power supply. In this case an inverter unit produces mains a.c. voltage from a car-type battery which is permanently on trickle charge from the normal mains supply. Failure of this causes the inverter to operate for as long as the battery lasts.

15.4 The use of radiofrequencies

The risk of a patient receiving an electric shock becomes negligible with currents of a few milliamperes at frequencies of some 20 kHz or higher. Thus, devices such as electrical impedance cardiographs and pneumographs which employ electrodes located on the thorax employ excitation frequen-

Figure 15.1 Rigel Model 255
Electrical Safety Tester.
(Courtesy Graseby Medical Ltd.)

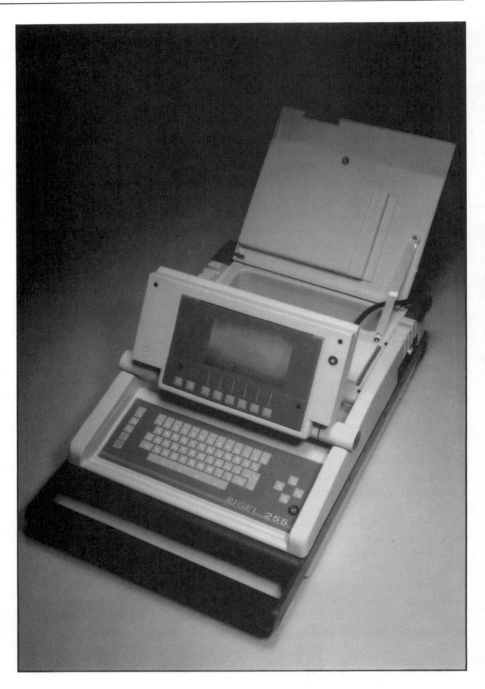

cies in the range 20 kHz to 100 kHz.

In the electrical impedance method for the monitoring of stroke volume
and cardiac output on a beat-by-beat basis, a current of some 4 mA r.m.s.
at 100 kHz is passed through the thorax via band electrodes placed around
the neck and around the bottom of the thorax at the level of the xiphis-

ternal joint. At each of these locations a separate band electrode picks up the voltage at 100 kHz developed by the constant current of 4 mA flowing through the chest. This voltage is proportional to the resistance of the thorax at 100 kHz. In an adult with normal lungs it is approximately 25 ohms and decreases by about 0.2 ohms transiently with each heart beat expelling blood into the aorta. From a knowledge of this reduction, the resistance of the thorax, the distance between the pick-up electrodes and the resistivity of the patient's blood, it is possible to calculate an approximate value for the stroke volume. Multiplying this by the heart rate yields the cardiac output.

Northridge, D. B., Finlay, J. N., Wilson, J., Henderson, E. and Dargie, H. J. (1990) 'Non-invasive determination of cardiac output by Doppler echocardiography and electrical bioimpedance', *British Heart Journal*, **63**, 93–7, compare two non-invasive methods used in intensive care units for cardiac output monitoring.

15.5 Electrical burns to the patient

15.5.1 Burns from d.c. supplies

Direct current is capable of producing nasty burns under electrodes on a patient's skin. Metal ions from the electrode may be driven into the skin by electrolysis. Devices connected to a patient should be incapable of passing more than 10 microamperes d.c. into the patient. Burns have been reported with only 3 volts d.c. involved.

15.5.2 Radiofrequency burns

The use of a surgical diathermy unit on a patient connected to monitoring equipment can give rise to serious radiofrequency burns which are slow to heal if the unit's plate electrode is not making a good contact with the patient, has not been placed in position or the lead to the plate is broken. Diathermy burns have occurred regularly in operating rooms but tend not to be discussed in wider circles.

15.6 Fires and explosions

The use of flammable anaesthetic agents such as ether and cyclopropane has now virtually ceased with the widespread use of modern non-inflammable agents. However, many operating rooms and anaesthetic rooms are still provided with anti-static electricity precautions which include conducting terrazzo floors and anti-static rubber tyres for trolley wheels and anaesthetic system rubber hoses.

Static electric charges can easily be induced on insulated metal objects in a dry atmosphere by friction and can then give rise to a micro-spark which can detonate anaesthetic mixtures of ether or cyclopropane in air or oxygen. Charges built up on trolleys or metal components linked to the anaesthetic machine via corrugated hoses can be leaked to earth or the conducting floor via rubber hoses and tyres made of conducting rubber. The resistance of a 1.5 metre length of corrugated hose should lie between 25 k ohms and 1 megohm while that of a trolley-wheel tyre should lie between 0 and 10 k ohms. This is sufficiently low that it will allow a static charge to leak away, but sufficiently high that it will not allow sufficient mains current to flow which might subject the patient to the risk of an electric shock.

Electrostatic charge can also build up on personnel with dry skin and shoes with insulating soles arising from friction between the body and manmade fibre underwear. Electric charge can only reside on the outside surface of a hollow electrically conducting surface. By wearing a gown or 'scrub suit' made of a porous cotton material which absorbs atmospheric water vapour, any charge present is conducted down to the terrazzo floor via the conducting soles of rubber boots or overshoes. The electrical capacity of the capacitor formed by the floor and earth is sufficiently large that charge accumulation on it does not raise the voltage to the extent at which a micro-spark can occur.

A zone of risk extends 25 cm in all directions around tubing carrying flammable anaesthetic mixtures. Equipment used inside this zone must be designed to be explosion-proof to the requirements of British Standard 5724. Conventional patient-monitoring equipment is used mounted on a shelf attached to, for example, an anaesthetic machine, so that it is more than 25 cm distant from the anaesthetic circuit.

Mixtures of ether and methylated spirit are often employed to clean the patient's skin at the site of operation and these can easily soak into the sterile drapes used to cover the patient. The mixture can be set on fire when cautery is used to seal bleeding points or by sparking within the quiver attached to the operating table which stores the diathermy cutting electrode when the diathermy unit is inadvertently activated by the surgeon accidently stepping on the footswitch. Health Circular (Hazard) (90)25, 19 June 1990, 'Ignition of spirit-based skin cleaning fluid by surgical diathermy setting fire to disposable surgical drapes resulting in patient burns' from the UK's Department of Health Medical Devices Directorate recommends that spirit-based fluids should not be used for skin cleaning, disinfection or preparation of patients for operations involving surgical diathermy. This is particularly important when other easily ignitable materials such as disposable drapes are in use. When the use of spirit-based fluids is unavoidable, it is important to ensure that the pooling of fluid does not occur and that the drapes do not become soaked. The fluid must be used sparingly and sufficient time allowed for the fluid to evaporate and the skin to dry before the diathermy is operated.

Apart from the risk of burns to the patient the discovery and subsequent extinguishing of smouldering drapes considerably upsets the routine of the operating team. 'Preventing, preparing for and managing surgical fires', *Health Devices*, **21**, 24–30, January (1992) states that the most obvious and easiest method of fighting fires is to prevent them starting! For a fire to be self-sustaining, heat, fuel and an oxidizer must come together in the correct proportions. If any of these elements can be reduced or eliminated the fire can be prevented or extinguished. Some possible sources of heat in the operating room include defibrillators, surgical diathermy and cautery and surgical lasers. Fuels include alcohol, degreasing agents such as ether and acetone, linens, dressings, aerosols and ointments, gloves, anaesthetic-system components, blood-pressure cuffs and disposable packing materials. Oxygen is the most commonly available oxidizer. One hundred per cent oxygen increases fire hazards compared with air. Stringent fire precautions are essential when patients are being treated in hyperbaric chambers. Flash fires can occur in the sealed chamber with devastating results and the pressurized chamber makes an emergency evacuation difficult.

Quite apart from the dangers arising from the heat of a fire, the combustion of plastic items can generate toxic smoke containing substances such as hydrogen chloride and fluoride, cyanide, phenol, aldehydes and complex hydrocarbons leading to asphyxiation. Operating room staff should 'Think the unthinkable' and prepare a fire plan involving action to be taken to disrupt and localize the fire, the correct use of fire extinguishers, the location of gas supply, heating and ventilation controls and of the fire alarm and communication system.

15.7 Cross-infection hazards

Items such as blood-pressure transducers, endoscopes and ventilators come into contact with patients' blood and secretions and, because of their expense, have to be shared among many patients. It is important that either the parts which come into contact with body fluids are 'one trip' disposable devices or that sterilization/disinfection of them is performed rigorously according to the manufacturer's instructions.

Commonly encountered chemical disinfection agents are formaldehyde and glutaraldehyde which are contained respectively in the commercial products Gigasept and Cidex. The maximum exposure limit of formaldehyde in the UK is two parts per million and for glutaraldehyde it is only 0.2 parts per million. These solutions must be used in well-ventilated conditions to prevent inhalation by staff. Mobile disinfection stations are available for use with items such as flexible endoscopes which contain fibre optics and miniature television camera chips. The air ventilated from the disinfection units passes through an active charcoal filter to ensure the removal of vapours and droplets.

Disposable blood-pressure transducers are available, but more commonly a disposable cuvette or 'dome' fitted with a slack plastic diaphragm can be easily connected on top of the silicon or metal diaphragm of the transducer's body. Disposable breathing hoses and connectors simplify the disinfection of ventilator circuits and must be disposed of via authorized routes.

Autoclaving is the best approach to sterilization but will cause irreparable damage to items such as blood-pressure transducers and fibre optic endoscopes. In these situations liquid chemical techniques or ethylene oxide gas or formalin vapour must be used with an adequate time cycle.

In order to prevent the airborne transmission of bacteria between ventilated patients in a hospital unit, high efficiency pleated membrane bacterial filters should be fitted to both the inspiratory and the expiratory ports of each ventilator. The filter elements are disposable and have been tested for particle penetration to the requirements of British Standard 3928. The filter fitted to the expiratory port is mounted in an electrically heated housing in order to prevent condensation of water from the patient's breath and should be changed for each patient. The inspiratory port filter should be replaced at intervals of approximately two months.

Equipment used with patients, which may have become infected, must be properly disinfected before service engineers are allowed access to repair it with a formal documented 'permission to work' system in operation to supervize the hand-over arrangement. For some surgical procedures, as in orthopaedics, it is necessary to have an 'ultra clean' operating room. In one arrangement, filtered air from a ventilating canopy in the ceiling is ducted downwards in the centre of the microbiologically clean zone which encompasses the operating table and its immediate surroundings which include the operating team and their instruments. The airflow is downwards at the centre of the zone and radially outwards at the periphery. Suction is also available from the system via lightweight tubes and snap-in connections. It is used in conjunction with operating gowns and extraction helmets or neck-loops to control the body emissions of the surgical team and prevent these contaminating the site of the operation. The constant upward flow of air within the gown makes it comfortable to wear and helps to reduce fatigue. Patient monitors, diathermy and ventilators are bathed in the downward flow of clean air sweeping away from the patient so that any emissions from the equipment would be cleared away by the ventilation system of the operating room.

Special flooring material for the entrance to operating room and intensive care areas is available which is designed to trap and retain dust particles on the wheels of trolleys which may carry harmful bacteria. It contains a bactericide, is easy to clean and has a life expectancy of two to three years. Wall-cladding materials are also available impregnated with a bactericide and suitable for use in operating theatres and intensive care units.

15.8 Mechanical hazards

Equipment used with patients should be the subject of regular planned preventative maintenance inspections with the object of detecting and correcting incipient faults. These might include bolts which have worked loose or not been replaced during a previous service, or parts which exhibit significant corrosion, cracking or deformation resulting in a weakness which could lead to a collapse. A collapsing patient head support has caused an elderly patient to fall on to the floor when an X-ray table was tilted into the head-down position. A power driven X-ray tube head attempted to crush the patient when a faulty micro-switch allowed the motor drive to unexpectedly start into action.

With routine wear and tear, quite apart from any faulty design, components can fail or become loose and constitute a risk to patients. The constant washing-over of metal parts with saline irrigation fluids can cause metal parts to be weakened by corrosion, and rusting can weaken steel cables. It has been reported that a senior anaesthetist was forced to take premature retirement consequent upon fracturing the neck of his femur after tripping over a trailing electric cable in an operating room. Retractable ceiling-mounted pendants are available for use in operating rooms and which provide several mains electrical outlets, suction and anaesthetic gases. Tubing and cables lead down to the equipment concerned, leaving the floor uncluttered, Figure 15.2.

15.9 Alarms

Patient monitors and the more sophisticated ventilators are usually fitted with alarm facilities to draw attention by means of audible and visual signals to the presence of conditions such as loose or disconnected electrodes, high or low heart and respiratory rates and high or low inflation pressures. These warnings can be most helpful, but do not substitute for regular contact with, and visual observation of the patient. It is important that the alarm cannot be cancelled only at a central station but at the bedside so that the patient is seen in relation to the alarm condition. The use of a double criteria (e.g. a tachycardia alarm not being activated unless it derives from both the ECG and a finger photoplethysmographic finger sensor) can minimize the prevalence of false alarms which irritate the staff and bring the system into disrepute.

15.10 Equipment management systems

Life-support equipment should form a major part of a comprehensive hospital equipment management scheme which covers: the initial formal justification for the new/replacement item of equipment and the writing of a detailed specification of performance; the preliminary selection of suppliers to be invited to tender against the specification; competitive tendering, evaluation of tenders against written criteria and post-tender negotiations; acceptance tests; staff training; servicing (maintenance, repair and modification); expected lifetime; replacement policy; and finance policy-capital purchase or lease.

Each item of equipment should carry a label which identifies its part number in the scheme and the telephone number of the organization to

Figure 15.2 Ceiling-suspended operating room pendant providing gas, suction and electrical supplies and mounting for an anaesthetic machine, ventilator and patient monitor. (Courtesy Draeger Medical Ltd.)

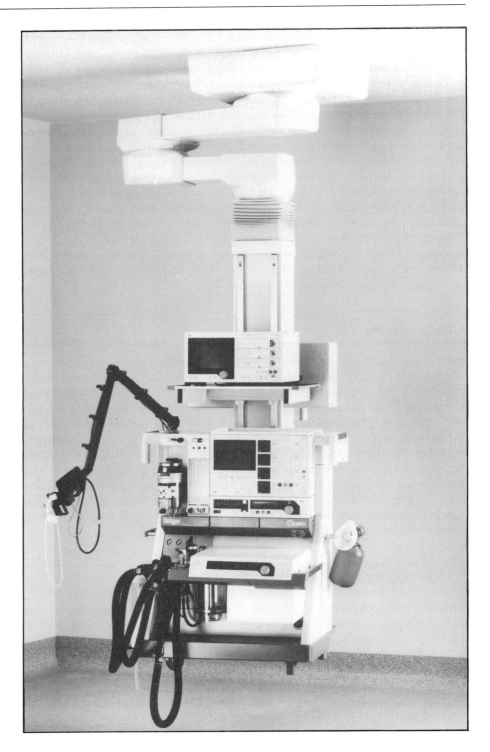

contact in the event of a problem arising with the equipment's function. Other distinctive labels should be used to indicate that modifications have been made or if the unit can be used on a limited basis pending the undertaking of further maintenance work. For example, it may be that a switch has stuck in the ON position and a replacement switch is not immediately available. It is possible to use the equipment with care, provided that the user is aware of the consequences of the switch being permanently ON.

Equipment for British hospitals should only be purchased from suppliers who feature on the UK Department of Health's Register of Manufacturers who operate agreed good manufacturing practices. The Department of Health published in November 1990 a booklet covering the 'Management of Medical Equipment and Devices' which sets out the elements of an equipment-management scheme for hospitals.

15.11 Safety at work considerations

So far, much of this chapter has been devoted to the safety of patients but it is also important to consider the safety of staff and visitors. In the UK the 1974 Health and Safety at Work Act provides the main legal framework and sets the minimum requirements for locations such as offices, factories and hospitals. It is an enabling Act which grants powers to introduce further detailed regulations as necessary. Most of the new safety legislation emanating from the European Communities is being introduced under this Act. In general, an employer must ensure 'so far as is reasonably practicable' the health, safety and welfare at work of all employees. Risks must be balanced against the cost of avoiding them. The Health and Safety Inspectorate regularly inspect hospitals and will require to see local safety documentation such as safety rules, authorization to work, staff records and to review the actions of safety representatives and safety committees.

With the removal of Crown Immunity from National Health Service hospitals, individual members of staff who are suspected of negligence in respect of unsafe products (which includes modifications and the use of devices built in-house) or procedures can be prosecuted and taken to court by the Health and Safety Inspectorate. Thus, in answering a possible prosecution, it is vital to have a well-documented scheme of work and to have followed correct procedures in the choice, operation and maintenance of equipment. The documentation must delineate the chain of management and the limits of each person's responsibilities.

New European Communities directives aimed at reducing the number of back injuries due to the manual handling of loads were added to the existing Health and Safety at Work Act at the start of 1993. The UK's Royal College of Nursing guidelines recommend that no individual should lift more than 30 kg unaided and that a hoist should always be used when lifting loads in excess of 50 kg. Emphasis is increasingly being placed on the provision of hoists and power-operated beds with adjustable bed height, backrests and knee-breaks. Electrically powered beds may feature three 24 V d.c. actuators to provide these movements and yet present no electrical hazard to the patient. A battery back-up can be provided to allow the patient and bed to be easily moved from one location to another.

Index